TAI CHI FOR SENIORS

Gentle 10-Minute Routines with Step-by-Step Illustrations & Video Guides to Prevent Falls, Ease Joint Pain, and Restore Strength, Balance & Independence

Table of Contents

INTRODUCTION

BEGINNING AGAIN WITH CONFIDENCE

Welcome: Reclaiming Ease at Any Age

The word "ease" carries weight as we grow older. It means more than simply moving without pain; it suggests moving with confidence, grace, and a sense of calm. For many people, aging feels like a gradual narrowing of what is possible. Simple actions like bending to tie a shoe, turning to greet someone behind you, or stepping off a curb can suddenly feel like calculated risks. The purpose of this book is not to ignore these realities, but to invite you to rediscover that movement can feel light, safe, and even enjoyable again.

Why Ease Matters More Than Speed or Strength

In younger years, exercise often revolves around pushing limits—running faster, lifting heavier, lasting longer. But research on older adults consistently shows that mobility and balance, not maximum strength, are the strongest predictors of long-term independence. For example, studies from the National Institute on Aging point to something as simple as walking speed being a marker of overall health in seniors. If you can walk at a steady pace without fear of stumbling, you are more likely to keep driving, cooking, and living on your own.

That is why tai chi is such a powerful tool. It is not about competing with anyone else or reaching athletic goals. Instead, it emphasizes balance, awareness, and controlled movement. These qualities feed directly into a life with less stress and fewer falls, which are among the greatest concerns for people in their sixties, seventies, and beyond.

Reframing What "Exercise" Means

The very word “exercise” often triggers resistance. For some, it brings back memories of intimidating gym classes or the thought of sore muscles and heavy breathing. Yet, exercise in later years does not need to resemble any of that. In fact, for many seniors, the best form of exercise looks more like play or meditation than traditional workouts.

Tai chi is sometimes described as “meditation in motion.” That phrase matters because it takes away the pressure of exercise as a chore. Instead of focusing on repetitions or heart rate, tai chi encourages you to notice how your feet press into the ground, how your breath fills the lungs, how your arms glide through the air. These details not only strengthen the body but also quiet the mind. For someone who may feel nervous about balance or stiff joints, this approach changes the narrative: movement becomes soothing rather than threatening.

Real Stories of Rediscovered Confidence

Consider a retired teacher who had given up gardening after a fall on her driveway. She started with just five minutes of simple tai chi arm movements while seated. Over weeks, she noticed her shoulders loosening and her breath deepening. Encouraged, she tried standing again, first with a hand on the counter, then unsupported. Months later, she returned to her flower beds, not because her pain had vanished completely, but because she trusted her body more.

Another example comes from a veterans’ community center in California, where tai chi classes have been offered for seniors with knee and hip replacements. Many participants reported that beyond physical balance, what kept them attending was the sense of calm they carried into the rest of the day. One man explained that he could finally sleep through the night without waking from anxiety, simply by repeating a breathing exercise before bed.

These accounts show that reclaiming ease is not about grand transformations but about small, steady wins.

The Mental Side of Ease

Physical comfort is only half the story. The fear of falling, or of looking weak in front of others, often becomes as limiting as actual aches and pains. When you hesitate to step off a bus or decline a walk with friends because of self-doubt, independence begins to shrink. Tai chi directly addresses this by pairing physical movement with mental focus. Each step, each shift of weight is intentional. This builds not just muscles, but confidence in your ability to handle daily life.

Psychologists who study aging note that confidence itself can prevent falls. When you believe you can catch yourself, you react faster and steadier. In this way, tai chi trains both body and mind to respond with calm rather than panic.

A Gentle Invitation

Reclaiming ease at any age begins with giving yourself permission to move again, slowly, gently, and without judgment. You do not need to perform perfectly, nor do you need to remember long sequences on the first try. The act of showing up, of breathing and shifting weight with awareness, is already progress.

Tai chi offers this invitation: to replace stiffness with flow, hesitation with trust, and fear with calm. Whether you are sixty-eight or eighty-five, whether you live with arthritis, high blood pressure, or just the natural changes of aging, ease is not a memory of youth. It is something you can cultivate right now, step by step, breath by breath.

What Tai Chi Can Do for Seniors (Balance, Joints & Brain)

Tai chi has been practiced for centuries, yet its power for modern seniors lies in how it touches three key areas that shape independence: balance, joint health, and brain function. These are often the first things people worry about as the years pass, and they are the very things this practice is designed to protect.

Balance: Standing Steady in a World That Moves

Falls are one of the greatest risks older adults face. According to the Centers for Disease Control and Prevention, about one in four seniors in the United States experiences a fall each year. The danger is not just the fall itself but the loss of confidence that follows. Many stop walking as much or avoid outings, which only makes muscles weaker and balance worse.

Tai chi directly trains the systems that keep you upright. Every slow step, weight shift, and pause forces your body to adjust. Unlike walking in a straight line, tai chi asks you to move diagonally, twist gently at the waist, or rise onto the ball of your foot. These small challenges teach your inner ear, eyes, and muscles to work together again.

A clinical study published in the *Journal of the American Geriatrics Society* showed that seniors practicing tai chi three times a week cut their risk of falling almost in half compared to those doing standard stretching. That is a dramatic change, not from jumping or sprinting, but from moving with attention and patience. Imagine how much peace of mind comes from knowing you can step off a curb without fear.

Joints: Moving Without Grinding or Strain

Arthritis, stiffness, and past injuries are familiar companions for many seniors. Traditional exercise can sometimes make these worse. Tai chi, by contrast, was designed to be low-impact. Movements are slow, knees stay softly bent, and there are no sudden jolts. You are always in control of how far to step, how deeply to bend, or how high to raise an arm.

Think of it as oiling the hinges rather than forcing them. Gentle repetition increases circulation to cartilage and connective tissues, which helps reduce stiffness. A woman recovering from hip replacement once shared that tai chi was the only activity she could do without feeling sharp pain afterward. Over time, she not only regained mobility but also noticed her posture improving because her muscles were supporting her joints better.

Medical groups such as the Arthritis Foundation recommend tai chi for this very reason. It strengthens the muscles around joints without pounding on them. If you wake up with creaky knees or sore shoulders, this practice offers a way to move that soothes instead of aggravates.

Brain: Sharpening Focus and Calming the Mind

Physical health is only one side of aging. Memory lapses, brain fog, and stress weigh just as heavily. Tai chi addresses this through its demand for mental focus. You cannot go on autopilot while practicing. You must remember the sequence, stay aware of your body, and sync your breath with each motion. This combination stimulates the brain in ways that crossword puzzles or television cannot.

Researchers at Harvard Medical School have reported that older adults practicing tai chi showed improvements in memory and executive function—skills needed for planning, decision-making, and attention. The rhythm of breathing and movement also lowers stress hormones, which supports better sleep and clearer thinking.

Seniors often describe this mental side as the most surprising gift. A retired accountant once said that tai chi was like "turning down the static" in his head. Instead of worrying about medications, bills, or aches, he found himself absorbed in the simple act of shifting weight from one leg to the other. That calm carried into his daily life, making him more patient and less anxious.

The Combined Effect

When balance, joints, and brain health all improve together, the outcome is larger than the sum of its parts. You feel steadier on your feet, less trapped by pain, and more confident in your thinking. This does not mean problems vanish. Arthritis will not disappear, nor will tai chi guarantee you never lose balance again. But what it does offer is control—control over how you move, how you react, and how you care for your body.

Tai chi gives you a way to keep these three areas—balance, joints, and brain—working together instead of wearing down. It shifts the focus from what has been lost with age to what can still be strengthened, protected, and enjoyed.

How to Use This Book, Videos & Alternatives

This book has been designed to make tai chi both approachable and practical, especially for seniors who may feel unsure about where to begin. You will notice that each chapter builds on the last, and that the lessons are meant to be used in small, manageable steps. The goal is not to overwhelm you with information, but to guide you through a daily routine that feels safe, clear, and rewarding.

Following the Structure

The layout is simple: you start with background chapters that explain why tai chi matters, followed by a set of basic movements. From there, the program is divided into weekly routines. Each week introduces seven poses—one for each day—but you are not expected to learn them all at once. Think of the structure as a menu. Some days you may practice just two or three moves, other days you may go through the full sequence. Both approaches are perfectly fine.

By the end of four weeks, you will have a complete 15-minute practice you can repeat for as long as you like. If you prefer to stay with Week 1 for two or three weeks before moving forward, that is also encouraged. The idea is progress, not pressure.

Step-by-Step Photos and Large Print

Every exercise is supported with large-print instructions and step-by-step photos. Seniors often complain about small text and vague illustrations in other exercise books, so special attention was given here to clarity. You should be able to place the book on a chair, table, or stand and follow along without straining your eyes. Each movement is written in plain English, avoiding unnecessary technical terms.

Using the Videos

Printed instructions are helpful, but sometimes you may want to see how a movement flows from start to finish. That is where the videos come in. Each exercise includes a code you can scan with a phone or tablet. Once scanned, the video will play a short demonstration, allowing you to watch as many times as needed.

If scanning codes feels uncomfortable, there are alternatives. You can type in a simple website address printed below each code, which will take you directly to the same video. For readers who prefer not to use the internet at all, a DVD version is available separately so you can watch on a television or DVD player. This way, no matter your level of comfort with technology, you have an option that works.

Adjusting to Your Pace

You are not expected to remember every detail right away. The best approach is repetition. Practice one pose at a time until it feels familiar, then add another. Some readers find it helpful to place a bookmark on the current page and keep returning to it until the move feels natural. Others prefer to watch the video while reading the book, pausing as needed. Experiment until you discover what helps you learn best.

Practical Tips for Everyday Use

Think of this book as a partner in your daily routine. Leave it in a place where you will see it often, such as beside your favorite chair or on the kitchen table. Consistency comes more easily when the reminder is visible.

Some readers like to practice in the morning, using the routine as a gentle warm-up for the day. Others prefer evening, finding that it helps release tension before bed. There is no “right” time. What matters is that you show up for yourself regularly, even if only for five minutes.

When following along, pay attention to how your body feels. If a step causes discomfort, shorten the movement or return to a seated variation. Remember that tai chi is about balance and flow, not force. The most important rule is to move in a way that feels safe.

Building Confidence Through Choice

This book gives you freedom of choice. You can use only the written instructions, combine them with the videos, or rely on the DVD. You can practice standing, seated, or holding onto a support. You decide how long to practice and when to progress. Many seniors find this flexibility reassuring because it removes the fear of "failing" or falling behind.

The intent is to meet you where you are today, whether you are recovering from a surgery, dealing with arthritis, or simply wanting to feel more steady and calm. Over time, the combination of clear instructions, visual support, and flexible pacing allows you to grow in confidence. The program is not about perfection—it is about rediscovering trust in your body, one small step at a time.

Read Me First: Safety Checks, Medications & When to Stop

Before starting any new activity, especially one involving movement and balance, it is wise to pause and think about safety. Tai chi is gentle, but that does not mean it is free from risks. A few simple checks and clear boundaries can make your practice both safer and more enjoyable.

Talking with Your Doctor

The first step is to have an honest conversation with your healthcare provider. Bring up the idea of beginning tai chi and ask if there are any specific restrictions for you. Doctors can give valuable guidance if you live with conditions like arthritis, high blood pressure, osteoporosis, or heart disease. They may suggest avoiding deep bends, quick turns, or holding your breath too long.

For example, a cardiologist might reassure you that tai chi is safer than brisk treadmill workouts for someone with heart disease, but they may also recommend standing near a chair for extra support during the first few weeks. This kind of advice helps you practice with confidence rather than fear.

Knowing Your Medications

Medications can influence balance, energy, and coordination. Blood pressure pills sometimes cause lightheadedness when standing up quickly. Medications for anxiety or sleep can leave you drowsy. Even common pain relievers may dull sensations, making it harder to notice when a joint is under stress.

This does not mean you cannot practice tai chi—it simply means you should be aware of how your medications affect you. Try exercising at a consistent time of day so you learn how your body responds. If you notice patterns, such as dizziness after taking morning pills, shift your practice to later in the day. Always inform your doctor if side effects interfere with your ability to move safely.

Safety Checks Before Practice

Think of each practice session as beginning with a mini checklist:

- Is the floor clear of rugs, cords, or clutter?
- Are you wearing comfortable shoes or practicing barefoot on a safe surface?
- Do you have a sturdy chair, counter, or wall nearby for support if needed?
- Are you feeling steady, alert, and not overly tired?

These checks take less than a minute but greatly reduce the chance of slips or strain. Seniors who skip these steps often find themselves distracted or unsteady, which can undermine the very purpose of tai chi—building confidence.

When to Stop

One of the most important lessons is learning when to pause. Many of us grew up hearing "no pain, no gain," but that mindset does not apply here. Discomfort is a warning, not a badge of honor. Stop immediately if you feel sharp pain, sudden dizziness, chest pressure, or blurred vision. These signals should never be ignored.

There is also the quieter voice of fatigue. If you feel unusually drained, unable to focus, or frustrated, it is better to end the session early. Returning the next day refreshed is far more valuable than forcing yourself to continue while struggling. Tai chi is meant to support your life, not drain it.

Practicing with Conditions in Mind

Different health conditions may require special attention. If you live with arthritis, keep movements small and focus on smooth transitions rather than large ranges of motion. For those with osteoporosis, avoid deep forward bends or twisting with force. Seniors with diabetes should pay attention to blood sugar levels and avoid practicing on an empty stomach.

A real-world example comes from senior centers that teach tai chi to people with Parkinson's disease. Instructors encourage participants to keep a chair in front of them, not because the moves are too difficult, but because the support reduces fear. With that reassurance, participants move more freely and gain more from the practice.

Listening to Your Own Body

Finally, the most reliable safety guide is your own awareness. Over time, you will develop a sense of which movements feel nourishing and which feel risky. Tai chi trains this self-listening by slowing everything down. Each shift of weight, each breath, gives you the chance to check in with how you are doing.

If you respect those signals—resting when tired, modifying when stiff, pausing when unsure—you will not only protect yourself but also deepen your practice. Tai chi is not a race or a performance. It is a conversation between your body and your mind, and safety is the language that allows that conversation to continue.

CHAPTER 1

THE TAI CHI WAY—PRINCIPLES FOR SAFE, GENTLE MOVEMENT

The Five Essentials: Posture, Breath, Softness, Intent, Flow

Tai chi may look like a graceful dance from the outside, but what makes it truly powerful are the inner principles guiding each move. These are sometimes called the "Five Essentials," and they are the foundation for practicing in a way that feels safe, calming, and effective. By paying attention to posture, breath, softness, intent, and flow, you not only improve how you move but also how you feel in daily life.

Posture: Building a Steady Foundation

Posture is the starting point for every tai chi movement. In simple terms, it means standing in a way that allows your body to feel both relaxed and supported. Imagine a string gently pulling the crown of your head upward, lengthening the spine without stiffness. At the same time, your shoulders soften downward, your chest opens, and your knees stay slightly bent.

Good posture redistributes weight through your hips and legs instead of loading pressure onto the knees or back. This is particularly important for seniors with arthritis or joint replacements. A man recovering from a knee replacement once described how tai chi posture taught him to stand tall without locking his knees, which reduced his pain during daily tasks like grocery shopping.

Breath: Linking Body and Mind

Breathing is more than taking in air; it is the rhythm that sets the pace of your movements. In tai chi, the breath should be natural, never forced. Typically, you inhale as the body opens—lifting arms or stepping forward—and exhale as the body closes—lowering arms or shifting weight back.

This pattern does two things: it supplies muscles with oxygen and it calms the nervous system. Scientists studying tai chi have noted that slow, deep breathing lowers heart rate and blood pressure while also reducing anxiety. For many seniors, learning to coordinate breath with motion feels like discovering a built-in stress reliever. You may even notice your sleep improving when you carry these breathing habits into bedtime.

Softness: Releasing Unnecessary Tension

Softness does not mean weakness. It means letting go of tight, rigid effort. If you have ever tried to open a jar with every muscle clenched, you know how tiring that approach can be. Tai chi teaches the opposite: use only the strength you need, and release the rest.

For someone with stiff shoulders, this can feel like a revelation. One woman in her seventies shared that she had been holding her shoulders up by her ears for decades without realizing it. Through tai chi, she learned to soften her upper body while keeping her legs strong. Not only did her shoulder pain decrease, but she also felt lighter and less fatigued throughout the day.

Softness also helps protect joints. Instead of locking elbows or pushing against resistance, movements are rounded and forgiving. This allows seniors to practice safely even when living with arthritis or chronic pain.

Intent: Moving with Awareness

Intent refers to the focus you bring to each action. Tai chi is not about waving your arms aimlessly; every gesture has purpose. When you extend your hand forward, imagine you are gently pushing away a curtain. When you shift weight to one foot, picture yourself rooting into the earth like a tree. These images help direct energy and sharpen concentration.

Studies on brain health show that this type of mindful movement improves memory and attention. Unlike automatic exercise machines, tai chi demands awareness, and that awareness keeps the mind sharp. For seniors worried about memory loss, this mental training is as valuable as the physical benefits.

Flow: Connecting It All Together

The final element, flow, ties posture, breath, softness, and intent into one continuous experience. Instead of jerky starts and stops, tai chi moves like water—smooth, unbroken, and calm. Think of a river moving around rocks: it doesn't freeze or fight, it simply adapts and keeps going.

Practicing flow teaches your body to transition gracefully between positions, which is exactly what is needed in daily life. Getting out of a chair, turning to reach for something, or stepping off a curb are all transitions. The smoother those transitions, the less chance of losing balance.

Flow also brings joy into the practice. Many seniors find themselves smiling after a session because the movements feel beautiful, almost like a gentle dance. It becomes less about "working out" and more about enjoying the sensation of moving freely again.

Putting the Essentials Together

Each of these five essentials—posture, breath, softness, intent, and flow—can stand on its own. But when practiced together, they transform tai chi from a set of exercises into a way of moving through life. Posture steadies the body, breath calms the heart, softness protects the joints, intent sharpens the mind, and flow connects everything in harmony.

By returning to these principles again and again, you will not only strengthen your tai chi practice but also rediscover ease in the simple acts of daily living.

Body Maps: Center of Gravity, Weight Shifts &

Joint-Friendly Range

Tai chi often looks effortless, but underneath the flowing movements lies a careful awareness of how the body carries weight. Understanding your center of gravity, learning to shift weight smoothly, and respecting the natural range of your joints are what make the practice safe and effective. For seniors, this awareness can be the difference between feeling wobbly and feeling steady.

Center of Gravity: Your Inner Anchor

Think of your center of gravity as the invisible point where your body balances. For most adults, it sits just below the navel, deep in the pelvis. As long as this point stays supported over your feet, you are stable. When it drifts too far outside that base—leaning forward while reaching for a shelf, or twisting quickly without support—the chance of losing balance rises.

Tai chi teaches you to keep your movements connected to this anchor. Instead of swinging arms wildly or stepping without thought, every gesture begins from the center. This creates a grounded feeling, much like the stability you feel when planting both feet firmly before lifting a heavy box. Seniors who practice with this awareness often notice they stop tripping as much or stumbling when turning in tight spaces.

An example comes from balance studies in rehabilitation clinics. Therapists found that patients who learned to consciously lower their center of gravity, even slightly, were far less likely to lose balance during daily activities. Tai chi naturally trains this ability, helping you feel secure when standing, walking, or reaching.

Weight Shifts: Learning the Art of Transition

Most falls happen not while standing still, but during transitions—stepping off a curb, pivoting to sit down, or turning to answer a call. Shifting weight without awareness can feel like lurching from one leg to the other. Tai chi replaces this with smooth, intentional transfers of weight.

When you shift in tai chi, you do it slowly. The heel comes down softly, the weight slides from one foot to the other, and the torso follows in harmony. Practicing this teaches your body to manage momentum, so you are never caught by surprise.

In one senior center program, instructors noted a sharp drop in falls among participants after six months of tai chi. The key was not strength gains alone, but the ability to sense when weight was moving forward or backward and adjust before it became a stumble.

A practical way to test this is at home: stand with feet shoulder-width apart and slowly move weight into one foot while keeping the other just lightly touching the floor. Notice the moment balance begins to feel uncertain. This kind of awareness is exactly what tai chi strengthens.

Joint-Friendly Range: Moving Without Strain

Joints—knees, hips, shoulders—often carry the scars of a lifetime of use. Arthritis, injuries, or surgeries can make wide movements painful. Pushing beyond a safe range not only hurts but may also increase the risk of falls. Tai chi solves this by encouraging motion in gentle arcs rather than forced extremes.

For example, instead of squatting deeply, tai chi uses soft knee bends where the thighs never move past a comfortable angle. Instead of swinging arms overhead, movements rise only to shoulder height unless more feels safe. This protects cartilage and ligaments while still encouraging circulation and flexibility.

The Arthritis Foundation has long recommended tai chi because of this principle. Studies show that participants practicing within joint-friendly ranges report less stiffness and greater ease in daily movements like climbing stairs or getting in and out of a car.

A retired nurse once described how tai chi taught her to "move like water around rocks." When her knees resisted deep bends, she simply flowed around the limitation, focusing on smaller arcs that still kept her active and pain-free.

Connecting the Three

When you bring these elements together—staying anchored in your center of gravity, shifting weight smoothly, and respecting joint-friendly ranges—you create a map of safe movement for your body. This map extends beyond practice sessions. It shapes how you stand in line at the grocery store, how you step into the shower, and how you turn to hug a grandchild.

Instead of fearing each step, you begin to recognize patterns: how your weight moves, where your center sits, and when your joints are asking for kindness. With time, these lessons become second nature, transforming tai chi into more than an exercise—it becomes a way of moving through daily life with steadiness and ease.

Pain vs. Progress: Listening to Your Body

One of the greatest challenges in later life is learning to distinguish between pain and the discomfort that comes with healthy progress. Tai chi invites you to move, but it also asks you to pay attention. The difference between listening and ignoring your body can determine whether this practice helps you feel younger or leaves you feeling discouraged.

Understanding the Signals

Pain is your body's alarm system. It is sharp, sudden, or persistent, often signaling that something is wrong. Progress, on the other hand, may feel like mild stretching, warmth in the muscles, or the slight fatigue that follows gentle exertion. The two sensations can sometimes be confused, especially if you are returning to movement after a long pause.

Take the example of knee arthritis. When you bend slightly in tai chi, you might feel stiffness as the joint wakes up. That stiffness may ease as you continue moving and should not leave you worse off later in the day. But if you feel stabbing pain that lingers or swells after practice, that is a warning sign. Knowing the difference allows you to continue with confidence instead of fear.

The Role of Gentle Stress

Muscles and joints adapt when they are challenged. Even in your seventies, your body responds positively to activity that nudges it beyond what is familiar. Physical therapists often refer to this as "progressive loading." In simpler terms, if you never ask your muscles to do a little more, they gradually weaken.

Tai chi provides that "little more" without the risks of heavy lifting or pounding movements. Shifting weight from one leg to the other, for instance, gently stresses the hip and thigh muscles. Over time, those muscles grow stronger, protecting the joints. A retired teacher once said she realized tai chi was working when climbing stairs became easier, not because her pain was gone, but because her legs were supporting her better.

Red Flags to Respect

There are clear signs that you should stop or modify what you are doing.

- Sharp or stabbing pain that does not ease with rest.
- Swelling or redness around a joint after practice.
- Dizziness, nausea, or blurred vision while moving.
- Chest pressure or sudden shortness of breath.

These are not signs of healthy progress. They are warnings to pause and, if necessary, consult your doctor. Respecting these limits is not weakness—it is wisdom.

Adjusting Instead of Quitting

Listening to your body does not mean giving up at the first sign of discomfort. It means making smart adjustments. If standing movements strain your knees, try the seated versions included in this book. If balance feels shaky, hold onto a sturdy chair. If you are short of breath, slow the pace and focus only on breathing with the arms.

One man recovering from back surgery found he could not twist at the waist without pain. Instead of abandoning practice, he focused on the upper-body moves until his core grew stronger. Months later, he reintroduced gentle waist turns without issue. His progress came not from ignoring pain, but from respecting it and finding another path forward.

Training Awareness

Perhaps the greatest gift of tai chi is that it trains awareness itself. By moving slowly, you notice small signals that might be overlooked in faster exercise. You learn how far you can step before the ankle complains, or how deeply you can bend before the hip resists. With practice, you become fluent in your body's language.

Researchers studying fall prevention have observed that seniors who practice tai chi often report fewer accidents not only because their muscles are stronger but because they are more aware of their limits. They sense when a step feels unsafe and adjust in time, rather than pushing through blindly.

Reframing Progress

Progress in tai chi is not measured in how many moves you memorize or how long you can stand on one leg. It is measured in smaller, subtler victories: waking up with less stiffness, catching yourself more smoothly when you stumble, feeling calmer after practice. These gains may not be flashy, but they are real and lasting.

By learning to separate pain from progress, you give yourself permission to move without fear. You stop chasing the exercise ideals of youth and instead build a practice that supports the body you have today. This balance—between listening and challenging—is what keeps tai chi safe, effective, and deeply rewarding for seniors.

Simple Self-Tests to Track Balance & Mobility

One of the best ways to stay motivated in tai chi is to see your progress over time. You may not notice small changes day to day, but with simple self-tests you can measure improvements in balance and mobility. These tests are not complicated, require no special equipment, and can be done safely at home. They give you real evidence that your practice is working.

The Sit-to-Stand Test

This test measures lower body strength and stability, both of which are directly linked to fall prevention. Sit in a sturdy chair with your arms crossed over your chest. Without using your hands, stand up and then sit back down. Time how many times you can do this in 30 seconds.

Most seniors find the first attempt a little challenging, but with practice, the number increases. Physical therapists often use this test to predict independence: the ability to rise from a chair without help is strongly tied to living on your own. If at first you can only manage two or three repetitions, do not be discouraged. Even one more the following week shows progress.

The Single-Leg Stand

Standing on one foot may sound simple, but it is a powerful way to gauge balance. Place a sturdy chair or counter nearby for safety. Lift one foot a few inches off the floor and hold as long as you can. Repeat on the other side. Record the time for each leg.

In research conducted by the National Institute on Aging, adults who could hold a single-leg stand for more than 10 seconds were less likely to experience falls. If your first attempt feels wobbly, that is normal. Tai chi directly trains the small stabilizing muscles in the ankles and hips that make this test easier over time.

The Step Test

Mobility is not just about standing still—it is about how quickly and safely you can move. The step test is simple: stand facing a low step, such as the bottom stair, and place one foot fully on it, then return it to the floor. Repeat this as many times as you can in 15 seconds, then switch legs.

This test measures coordination, agility, and leg strength. It also mimics daily life, like stepping off a curb or climbing onto a bus. Improvement in this test often translates directly into confidence outdoors. One senior in a community class shared that after practicing tai chi for two months, she felt steadier getting on her porch steps without needing to grip the railing.

The Reach Test

Balance often fails not when standing tall but when reaching out. The reach test helps you measure how stable you are when extending forward. Stand with feet shoulder-width apart and raise one arm straight ahead at shoulder height. Keeping your feet flat, reach forward as far as possible without stepping or losing balance. Measure the distance.

Falls often occur when someone leans too far outside their base of support. Practicing tai chi, which trains controlled weight shifts, gradually increases your reach distance. Over time, you may find that you can comfortably reach for items on a high shelf or bend forward without fear of toppling.

Tracking Results

These tests are not about competition with others. They are about comparing you to yourself. Keep a small notebook or use a calendar to record your times and repetitions every few weeks. Even modest improvements—an extra second of balance, one more chair rise—represent real gains in strength and safety.

Researchers often say, "what gets measured gets managed." By tracking these numbers, you remind yourself that small steps add up. A woman in her late sixties once commented that while she still felt stiff in the mornings, her notebook showed her single-leg balance doubled over three months. That simple fact gave her confidence to keep practicing.

Staying Safe While Testing

Always perform these tests near support, such as a wall, counter, or sturdy chair. Do not test when you are overly tired, dizzy, or recovering from illness.

If any test feels unsafe, skip it and return another time. The purpose is awareness, not pushing beyond limits.

By using these simple checks, you create your own scorecard of balance and mobility. They remind you that tai chi is not only about graceful movements in the moment—it is also about building steady, measurable improvements that support your independence every day.

CHAPTER 2

BALANCE & FALL-PREVENTION TOOLKIT

Your Base of Support: Stances That Keep You Steady

When it comes to preventing falls, one of the simplest but most powerful concepts is the base of support. Think of it as the foundation of a house: the wider and stronger it is, the less likely the structure is to topple. For your body, the base of support is created by your feet and how you place them on the ground. Tai chi emphasizes stances that make you more stable and better able to handle unexpected shifts in balance.

Why the Base of Support Matters

Every time you walk, stand, or even reach for something, your body relies on the size and position of your base. The wider your feet are apart, the more stable you become, but too wide a stance can make moving awkward. On the other hand, standing with your feet very close together makes it easier to topple, especially if someone bumps you or you lose concentration.

Research on falls in older adults consistently shows that most accidents occur during transitions—getting out of a chair, stepping off a curb, or turning quickly. A stable stance not only makes these transitions safer but also reduces the strain on your joints. By practicing stances in tai chi, you retrain your body to instinctively find positions that protect you from losing balance.

The Natural Stance

This is where many tai chi practices begin. Stand with feet about shoulder-width apart, toes pointing forward, and knees slightly bent. Your weight is spread evenly between both legs, with shoulders relaxed and arms hanging gently at your sides.

The natural stance may not look like much, but it builds awareness. Many seniors discover that they habitually lock their knees or lean slightly forward without realizing it. By correcting these habits, the body learns to distribute weight evenly, which reduces the risk of tipping when moving.

The Bow Stance

The bow stance is one of the most common positions in tai chi. Imagine standing with one foot forward and the other back, as if preparing to take a step. The front knee bends slightly while the back leg stays straight but relaxed. Your weight shifts mostly to the front leg, but not so much that you feel unsteady.

This stance trains you to handle forward and backward motions safely. It mimics the act of stepping off a curb or walking uphill, where most of the weight is temporarily on one leg. Practicing the bow stance teaches your body how to remain grounded during these everyday challenges.

The Horse Stance

Picture sitting on a tall, invisible stool with feet placed wider than shoulder-width apart, knees bent slightly, and torso upright. This is the horse stance. It builds leg strength and stability without requiring sudden movement.

For seniors, this stance is particularly useful for training the muscles that support the hips and knees. Stronger leg muscles mean more stability in daily life, whether it's rising from a chair or catching yourself after a misstep. A senior group in Florida once reported that practicing horse stance for just a few minutes daily helped participants feel steadier while gardening or shopping.

The Empty Stance

In the empty stance, most of your weight is on one leg while the other lightly touches the ground with the heel or toes. It may feel like a smaller version of balancing on one foot, but with extra support.

This stance teaches sensitivity. By practicing shifting almost all your weight to one side, you strengthen the stabilizing muscles in your hips and ankles. It also prepares you for movements where you must reach or step without fully committing your weight, such as testing the firmness of a step before walking across it.

Training with Awareness

The power of these stances does not come from holding them rigidly, but from practicing them with awareness. Tai chi is not about locking yourself into position; it is about finding balance in stillness and in motion. As you practice, notice how your feet feel against the floor. Are your toes gripping? Are your heels lifting? Are your knees stiff? Small adjustments often make a big difference.

In rehabilitation settings, therapists often teach patients recovering from hip surgery to imagine "triangles" under their feet, with weight spread between the heel and the ball of the foot. Tai chi stances naturally encourage this same balanced distribution.

Bringing Stances into Daily Life

These stances are not limited to practice sessions. They transfer directly into daily life. The natural stance is how you wait in line. The bow stance is how you step into a shower safely. The horse stance is how you reach down to pick up groceries without straining your back. The empty stance is how you test your footing on an uneven sidewalk.

By practicing them, you train your body to default to stability in moments when it matters most. Instead of feeling uncertain, your legs know how to position themselves, and your feet automatically widen your base of support when needed. That is the quiet strength tai chi builds—practical, steady, and ready to serve you every day.

Vision, Inner Ear & Feet—Training the Three Balance Systems

Balance may feel like a single skill, but in reality it is a partnership between three systems: your eyes, your inner ear, and your feet. Each one provides information to the brain, and together they decide whether you remain upright or take a tumble. As we age, one or more of these systems may weaken, but the good news is that they can all be trained and supported. Tai chi, with its focus on slow, deliberate movement, engages all three.

Vision: Seeing Stability

Your eyes are often the first line of defense for balance. They scan the environment, judge distances, and tell you if the ground ahead looks safe. But vision can be tricky. Poor lighting, cluttered rooms, or eye conditions such as cataracts or macular degeneration may interfere with what your brain perceives.

Tai chi helps by teaching you not to rely solely on vision. For instance, when you practice slowly shifting weight from one leg to the other, you are asked to feel the ground through your feet rather than constantly watching them. This reduces dependency on eyesight and trains other senses to compensate.

That said, vision is still vital. A practical step you can take is to keep rooms well lit, especially stairways and hallways. During tai chi, practice looking forward rather than down at your feet. This mimics real-world situations, like walking on a sidewalk, where your gaze must be ahead of you even as your feet adjust.

Inner Ear: The Silent Gyroscope

Hidden deep inside your skull is the vestibular system, a series of canals in the inner ear filled with fluid. As your head tilts or turns, that fluid shifts and sends signals to the brain about direction and speed. It is your body's silent gyroscope.

With age, this system can weaken, leading to dizziness or unsteadiness. Some medications also affect it. Tai chi supports the vestibular system by incorporating gentle head movements, controlled turns, and changes in direction. Unlike abrupt spins or quick pivots in other activities, these motions are slow, giving the inner ear time to adapt.

A striking example comes from fall-prevention studies in older adults with vestibular disorders. Those who practiced tai chi regularly reported fewer dizzy spells and greater confidence in crowded environments. They learned to recalibrate their sense of orientation through mindful movement.

Feet: Your Connection to the Ground

Your feet are loaded with nerve endings that act like sensors. They tell your brain whether you are standing on firm ground, soft carpet, or uneven gravel. Unfortunately, conditions like diabetes or neuropathy can dull this feedback, making it harder to adjust quickly when balance is challenged.

Tai chi emphasizes grounding through the soles of the feet. Each step is placed with awareness, and weight is shifted gradually, giving the brain time to register where the support lies. Even the simple act of rocking from heel to toe in practice strengthens the connection between feet and balance.

In one community program, seniors with foot numbness reported feeling safer walking outdoors after several weeks of tai chi. They explained that paying attention to the sensations they still had—pressure in the heels, the stretch of the arches—made them steadier despite reduced sensation.

Training All Three Together

What makes tai chi unique is that it engages vision, inner ear, and feet simultaneously. A slow turn to the side requires you to keep your eyes focused, your inner ear to track the rotation, and your feet to support the shift. Practicing this combination teaches the systems to work together, much like instruments in an orchestra. If one instrument falters, the others step in to keep the performance going.

You can try a simple exercise at home: stand in a natural stance, then close your eyes while gently swaying forward and back. Notice how your feet and inner ear take over when vision is removed. Add a slight head turn, and you are training all three systems at once. This exercise should always be done near a support, like a wall or sturdy chair, but it gives you a real sense of how balance depends on teamwork inside your body.

Everyday Applications

These balance systems are not just theory—they play a role in nearly everything you do. Crossing a busy street relies on vision. Turning your head to greet someone while walking tests your inner ear. Stepping onto a sandy beach challenges your feet. Tai chi prepares you for all these everyday demands by giving you practice in safe, controlled conditions.

The more you engage these three systems together, the better they will serve you in unpredictable situations. Whether you are walking through a dim restaurant, standing on a crowded bus, or navigating uneven ground, your training will help each system step up when needed. This is the quiet strength of tai chi: it conditions the body to stay steady not just in practice, but in the unpredictable rhythm of daily life.

Home Safety Walkthrough: Fall-Proofing Your Space

The safest tai chi practice starts not in the park or the studio, but in your own home. For many seniors, the house is both a sanctuary and a hazard. More than half of falls happen indoors, often in familiar rooms where clutter, poor lighting, or uneven flooring create hidden traps. A thoughtful walkthrough of your living space can dramatically reduce risks and make practicing—and daily life—more secure.

The Entryway

Falls often begin right at the doorstep. Wet shoes, uneven mats, or poorly lit porches can turn a welcome home into a danger zone. Choose a low-profile doormat that grips the floor rather than one with curled edges. If steps lead to your door, install sturdy railings on both sides and make sure lighting is bright enough to illuminate the entire path. Solar-powered lights along walkways are inexpensive and provide extra visibility at night.

One senior I worked with discovered that her favorite heavy rug at the entry was sliding on her hardwood floor. A simple rubber mat underneath stopped it from shifting and gave her peace of mind.

The Living Room

The living room is where many people trip, often because of clutter or furniture placed too closely together. Begin by clearing walkways. If cords or wires cross the room, secure them along the wall with covers. Rearrange furniture so there is a clear path wide enough for steady walking, even if you are carrying laundry or using a cane.

Consider replacing low coffee tables or footstools with something more stable. These items are easy to trip over and often overlooked. For tai chi practice, this room can become your training space, so keep an area clear where you can move freely without bumping into furniture.

The Kitchen

Kitchens combine movement, spills, and sometimes poor flooring. Keep items you use daily—like plates, cups, and pans—on shelves that are easy to reach without stretching or bending too far. Non-slip mats in front of the sink and stove protect against slipping on spilled water or grease.

Lighting is especially important in the kitchen. Under-cabinet lights make counters easier to see, reducing the chance of accidents with sharp tools. If bending to reach lower cupboards feels unstable, consider using pull-out drawers or baskets that bring items toward you rather than forcing you to crouch.

The Bedroom

It may feel like the safest room in the house, but many falls happen here when getting in or out of bed. Place a sturdy lamp or motion-activated nightlight near the bedside so you are never walking in the dark. Keep slippers with non-slip soles next to the bed, and avoid walking in socks on smooth floors.

Make sure your bed is the right height. If it is too high, you risk stumbling when climbing in. If it is too low, rising from it can strain your knees or hips. A supportive chair nearby can also help when dressing, allowing you to sit rather than balance on one foot.

The Bathroom

The bathroom is the most common site of indoor falls. Water, smooth tiles, and tight spaces create the perfect storm. Install grab bars near the toilet and inside the shower or bathtub. Do not rely on towel racks—they are not designed to hold weight.

Use non-slip mats both inside and outside the shower. A shower chair and handheld showerhead can add safety and comfort. If you prefer baths, consider a bath bench or a transfer seat that allows you to sit while getting in and out. Bright lighting in this room is critical; shadows can hide slippery spots.

Stairs and Hallways

Stairs are high-risk areas, especially if they are steep or uneven. Every staircase should have railings on both sides. Check that carpet runners are securely fastened, and avoid placing decorative items on steps.

Hallways should be kept clear of clutter and well lit. Motion-sensor nightlights placed along the baseboards can guide your way during nighttime trips to the bathroom.

General Tips for the Whole House

- Keep floors clear of loose rugs, or secure them with slip-resistant pads.

- Place phones or emergency alert systems in multiple rooms so you never feel pressured to rush.
- Wear supportive footwear indoors—slippers with sturdy soles are better than socks or bare feet.
- Regularly review your home setup. What felt safe last year may not fit your current needs.

A study by the CDC found that simple modifications—like better lighting, grab bars, and non-slip mats—reduced falls in older adults by nearly 40 percent. That is a significant number for such straightforward changes.

Your home should be a place where you feel steady and secure, not cautious and restricted. By taking the time to walk through each space with safety in mind, you create an environment where tai chi practice and daily activities become opportunities for strength, not risks for injury.

How to Recover from a Stumble: Step, Hip & Reach Strategies

Everyone stumbles. The difference between a small scare and a serious fall often comes down to how the body reacts in the split second after losing balance. Tai chi training gives you tools to respond calmly and effectively, rather than stiffening up or panicking. By practicing simple strategies—stepping, hip adjustments, and reaching—you can improve your ability to recover safely when life throws a wobble your way.

Step Strategies: Catching Yourself in Motion

The most natural reaction to a stumble is to take a step. The problem arises when the step is too short, too slow, or in the wrong direction. Tai chi helps by teaching deliberate, well-placed steps that keep your base of support under you.

Imagine tripping forward slightly. Instead of collapsing, your body needs to extend the front foot quickly and firmly, landing heel first, then rolling the weight through the foot. Tai chi's bow stance mirrors this motion, training you to shift weight smoothly onto the forward leg.

Backward stumbles can be harder, since most people rarely practice stepping back. Tai chi changes that by including controlled backward steps in many routines. Practicing these prepares you for real-life moments—like when you misjudge a chair behind you and need to step back quickly to avoid sitting in mid-air.

Studies on fall prevention consistently show that seniors who train reactive stepping are less likely to fall. In fact, a Canadian study found that practicing controlled steps in different directions reduced fall risk by almost 40 percent.

Hip Strategies: Shifting Your Center of Gravity

Sometimes, there isn't time for a big step. Instead, balance can be saved by moving the hips. Think of your hips as the steering wheel of your balance. If you lean too far to one side, a quick shift of the hips over the supporting leg can bring your center of gravity back into place.

Tai chi strengthens this response through constant weight-shifting exercises. Each time you move from one stance to another, your hips are quietly learning how to guide your weight safely. This not only builds muscle memory but also strengthens the core muscles around the waist and pelvis that provide stability.

One woman in her seventies shared how tai chi helped her when she slipped on a wet grocery store floor. Instead of falling sideways, she instinctively shifted her hips over her standing leg and caught herself. She described it as "the move my body remembered before my brain did."

Reach Strategies: Using the Upper Body Wisely

Reaching is often misunderstood in fall recovery. Reaching wildly can actually pull you off balance faster. But controlled reaching—using the arms to counterbalance or to steady yourself on nearby support—can prevent a fall.

Tai chi movements such as "Brush Knee" or "White Crane Spreads Wings" involve extending the arms with awareness while the lower body stays grounded. This trains coordination between upper and lower body, so the arms help restore balance instead of creating chaos.

A practical example: if you stumble sideways, extending the arm slightly in the opposite direction can counterbalance the shift. If there's a railing, countertop, or sturdy chair within reach, using the arms calmly to brace against it can turn a dangerous fall into nothing more than a stumble.

Practicing Recovery in a Safe Setting

You can practice these strategies at home in controlled ways. Stand near a sturdy counter or wall and practice taking larger-than-normal steps forward, backward, and sideways. Notice how your hips and arms naturally join the movement to steady you. Practice shifting your hips gently over one foot and then the other. Add arm movements that feel balanced rather than flailing.

It may feel odd at first to rehearse stumbles, but athletes have done it for years. Gymnasts, for example, train to fall safely so they can recover quickly. Seniors can use the same principle, practicing controlled reactions in a safe space until the body remembers how to respond under pressure.

Why Staying Relaxed Matters

Fear is often the biggest obstacle to recovery. When startled, the body tends to stiffen, which makes falls more likely. Tai chi's slow, mindful practice trains you to stay relaxed even during challenging movements. Over time, this calmness carries over into real-life stumbles. Instead of panicking, you respond with a clear, practiced action—step, hip shift, or reach.

CHAPTER 3
BREATH, CALM & MINDSET

Diaphragmatic Breathing Made Easy

Breathing is something you have done every day of your life, yet most people rarely think about how they breathe. Shallow breaths high in the chest become the default, especially during stress or as the posture stiffens with age. Diaphragmatic breathing—sometimes called belly breathing—reawakens the body's natural rhythm and brings calm while improving oxygen flow. The good news? It is far simpler than it sounds.

What the Diaphragm Does

The diaphragm is a dome-shaped muscle that sits just below the lungs. When you breathe in deeply, it contracts and flattens, creating space for the lungs to expand. When you breathe out, it relaxes, pushing air out gently. In early childhood, this is how everyone breathes, but by adulthood many people rely more on chest muscles, which are less efficient.

The difference is easy to feel. Place one hand on your chest and one on your abdomen. If only the chest hand rises with each breath, the diaphragm is not being used effectively. When the abdominal hand rises and falls smoothly, you are engaging the diaphragm.

Why It Matters for Seniors

As we age, lung capacity naturally decreases, and shallow breathing compounds the problem. Diaphragmatic breathing helps by maximizing the amount of oxygen taken in with each breath. It also stimulates the vagus nerve, which calms the heart rate and lowers blood pressure.

Doctors often teach this technique to patients recovering from surgery, heart conditions, or anxiety disorders. For seniors practicing tai chi, diaphragmatic breathing is more than a medical exercise—it is the engine that drives movement. A slow exhale can guide a graceful step, while a full inhale supports posture and energy.

Practicing the Technique

Start by sitting comfortably in a chair with your back supported and shoulders relaxed. Place one hand on your abdomen just below the ribs. Inhale slowly through the nose, noticing your abdomen expand outward like a balloon filling with air. Exhale through the mouth, letting the abdomen gently contract.

In the beginning, it may help to exaggerate the motion so you can feel it clearly. Once it becomes familiar, the movement will be more subtle. Practice for five minutes at a time, gradually increasing as it feels natural.

Some people worry that they are "doing it wrong" if they do not feel dramatic changes immediately. But remember, even small improvements in breathing depth provide real benefits over time.

Combining Breath with Movement

Tai chi offers a natural way to pair diaphragmatic breathing with physical motion. For example, as you slowly raise your arms outward, inhale gently, allowing the abdomen to expand. As you lower the arms, exhale fully, letting the abdomen contract. This synchronization creates flow between body and breath, making movements feel lighter and steadier.

One senior in a tai chi class described it this way: "When I focus on my breath, the movement feels like it's carrying me instead of me forcing it." This sense of effortlessness is one of the reasons diaphragmatic breathing has been practiced for centuries in martial arts and meditation.

Practical Everyday Uses

Beyond practice, diaphragmatic breathing can be a tool for daily life. Waiting at the doctor's office, dealing with restless nights, or calming nerves before a presentation to the community—all become easier with this simple technique.

A quick exercise: try breathing deeply for six slow cycles before bed. Many people find this helps them fall asleep faster and sleep more deeply. Others use it to reset after moments of stress, such as nearly tripping or feeling flustered in a crowded place.

Common Mistakes and Gentle Fixes

It is natural at first to tense the shoulders or force the breath. If you notice strain, pause and reset. The key is gentleness. The breath should feel like water flowing in and out, not like air being pumped. Another mistake is holding the breath unconsciously between inhales and exhales. Aim for a smooth, continuous rhythm, like a tide rolling in and out.

If lying down feels easier than sitting, practice in bed with knees bent and feet flat. This position naturally encourages the diaphragm to expand and can be particularly helpful for those with back discomfort.

Diaphragmatic breathing does not require perfection. It is less about performing correctly and more about rediscovering the body's natural rhythm. Each time you practice, even for a minute, you give your lungs, heart, and mind a moment of relief and reset.

Switch On the Relaxation Response in 60 Seconds

Stress is sneaky. It can show up as a tight jaw, stiff shoulders, or restless nights. Many seniors describe it as a low hum always running in the background. Fortunately, your body has a built-in reset button called the relaxation response, discovered in the 1970s by cardiologist Dr. Herbert Benson. This response is the opposite of the "fight-or-flight" mode—it slows the heart, lowers blood pressure, and calms the mind. And with the right practice, you can trigger it in about a minute.

What Happens in the Body

When stress hits, the sympathetic nervous system takes charge. Heart rate speeds up, breathing becomes shallow, and muscles tighten. The relaxation response activates the parasympathetic nervous system, slowing everything down. Think of it as flipping from the accelerator to the brake pedal. The change doesn't take hours of meditation. Research shows that even sixty seconds of focused breathing or gentle movement can start the shift.

The 60-Second Breath Reset

One of the simplest ways to activate the relaxation response is through breathing. Here's a technique you can try anywhere, even sitting in a waiting room:

- Sit comfortably and rest your hands on your lap.
- Inhale slowly through your nose for a count of four.
- Exhale gently through pursed lips for a count of six.
- Repeat this cycle for one minute.

By extending the exhale slightly longer than the inhale, you signal the nervous system to settle. Many people notice their shoulders dropping without even trying.

A retired accountant once shared that he used this technique before giving a speech at his granddaughter's wedding. "I went from shaking to smiling in less than a minute," he said.

Adding Gentle Movement

Tai chi adds another layer by pairing breath with slow, mindful movement. Even a simple exercise like lifting your arms with the inhale and lowering them with the exhale can create a wave of calm. This coordination keeps the mind anchored in the present, which quiets racing thoughts.

In a study on older adults, those who practiced short bouts of tai chi breathing and movement during the day reported less anxiety and fewer sleep problems compared to those who only rested quietly. The body seems to respond more strongly when breath and motion work together.

Using Focused Attention

Another way to trigger relaxation is by directing your attention. Instead of thinking about everything that went wrong today—or could go wrong tomorrow—choose a single word or phrase. Many people pick calming words such as "peace," "soft," or "quiet." With each exhale, repeat the word silently.

It may sound too simple to work, but repetition occupies the busy part of the brain and allows the body to shift gears. Think of it as giving your mind a soft handhold so it doesn't wander into worry.

Everyday Applications

The beauty of these techniques is that they are portable. You can use them while waiting for the kettle to boil, sitting in traffic, or lying awake at night. Stressful moments rarely give you thirty minutes to roll out a yoga mat, but they almost always give you sixty seconds to breathe, move, or focus.

Caregivers often find this especially useful. One woman caring for her husband with dementia practiced the 60-second breath reset whenever she felt overwhelmed. "It didn't solve everything," she admitted, "but it kept me from snapping when I was at the edge."

Building a Habit

The more you practice switching on the relaxation response, the quicker your body learns the pattern. At first, it might take the full minute to feel the shift. Over time, you may find calm settling in after just a few breaths. This conditioning is similar to muscle memory—it becomes easier the more often you repeat it.

Stress may be inevitable, but staying stuck in it is not. With breath, gentle movement, or focused attention, you have the ability to reset your nervous system in a surprisingly short amount of time.

Mindful Attention Without Sitting Still

When most people hear the word "mindfulness," they imagine someone sitting cross-legged, eyes closed, in perfect stillness. For many seniors, that picture is discouraging. Stiff hips, restless legs, or a wandering mind can make seated meditation feel like an impossible task. But mindfulness does not require stillness. In fact, tai chi shows that mindful attention can flourish while the body is in motion.

What Mindful Attention Really Means

At its core, mindfulness is simply paying attention to the present moment without judgment. Instead of reliving yesterday's arguments or worrying about tomorrow's errands, you notice what is happening right now. This could be the feel of your feet on the ground, the rhythm of your breathing, or the movement of your arms through space.

Research has confirmed that this kind of attention reduces stress, lowers blood pressure, and improves sleep. It even changes the way the brain processes pain, making discomfort easier to live with. And none of these benefits depend on sitting in silence for hours—they depend on noticing.

Tai Chi as Moving Mindfulness

Tai chi provides the perfect setting to practice mindfulness without stillness. Every slow, deliberate movement invites you to notice details: how your weight shifts from one leg to the other, how your shoulders relax, how your breath synchronizes with the motion.

For example, try lifting your arms as if floating them through water. Pay attention to the slight resistance in the air, the weight in your elbows, the sensation of your hands rising and falling. In this moment, the mind is fully anchored in the body. That is mindfulness in action.

One senior once joked, “I’m too fidgety to meditate, but when I’m doing tai chi, I sneak mindfulness in without realizing it.”

Everyday Mindfulness in Motion

Mindful attention does not need to be limited to formal practice. Walking down a hallway, you can notice the feel of each step. Washing dishes, you can focus on the warmth of the water and the sound of the plates. Even brushing your teeth can become mindful if you notice the sensation of the bristles and the rhythm of your breath.

This everyday approach has been studied in healthcare workers and caregivers, groups often under high stress. Those who practiced short, mindful moments during daily tasks reported less burnout and better mood. The same approach applies beautifully to older adults, especially those who feel frustrated by the idea of “traditional” meditation.

The Role of Breath in Moving Mindfulness

Breath acts as a bridge between body and mind. By pairing movement with diaphragmatic breathing, you create a natural rhythm that holds attention in the present. Inhale as you expand into a movement, exhale as you release. The breath cues the body, and the body cues the mind.

This is why many tai chi instructors emphasize breathing as much as posture. It is not just about oxygen; it is about giving the mind a simple anchor.

Practicing Without Pressure

Mindfulness sometimes gets sold as a cure-all, but that can add pressure: “If I can’t stay focused, I must be failing.” The truth is, the mind will wander. That is part of being human. The practice is not about keeping attention locked in place but about noticing when it drifts and gently returning it.

In tai chi, this happens naturally. Your attention may slip into daydreams, but the next shift of weight or arm movement calls you back. Over time, this repeated return strengthens awareness just as lifting weights strengthens muscles.

Why Moving Mindfulness Works for Seniors

For older adults, mindful movement has particular advantages. Sitting still too long can cause stiffness or discomfort, but gentle motion keeps joints warm and muscles active. It also feels purposeful—walking, swaying, or practicing tai chi movements has an immediate sense of "doing something," which makes the practice more engaging.

Researchers studying fall prevention note that mindful attention during movement may reduce accidents. By noticing weight shifts and body sensations in real time, seniors are less likely to be caught off guard by a stumble. Awareness becomes both calming and protective.

Mindful attention without sitting still offers a practical path: you do not have to be still to be present. You simply have to notice, in motion, what your body and breath are already doing.

Sleep Better: Evening Wind-Down with Tai Chi

Sleep can become elusive with age. Many older adults report falling asleep later, waking more often during the night, or rising earlier than they would like. Medications, chronic pain, or simply an overactive mind can all interfere. While sleep aids may offer temporary relief, research shows that gentle movement and breath practices are powerful, drug-free tools for improving rest. Tai chi provides an ideal evening wind-down, helping the body shift from daytime alertness to nighttime calm.

Why Sleep Changes with Age

Biologists point out that the body's internal clock, known as the circadian rhythm, shifts with age. Melatonin, the hormone that signals bedtime, is produced in smaller amounts. Add to this the muscle stiffness or aches that make it harder to find a comfortable sleeping position, and you have a recipe for restless nights. Stress and anxiety also play a role; the mind that races in the evening often drags the body along with it.

Tai chi addresses several of these issues at once. It reduces stress hormones, loosens tense muscles, and promotes the deep, diaphragmatic breathing linked to restful sleep.

The Evening Transition

The body needs cues to switch from “day mode” to “night mode.” In younger years, physical activity naturally provides this, but with age, activity levels often drop. Without that movement, the body may not receive a clear signal to slow down. A short tai chi session in the evening acts as a bridge: active enough to release tension, gentle enough not to overstimulate.

A practical example is a 15-minute routine of slow weight shifts, gentle arm circles, and deep breathing. Done consistently, this practice can become a signal to the body: it is time to let go and prepare for rest.

Calming the Nervous System

Tai chi activates the parasympathetic nervous system—the part responsible for relaxation and digestion. By combining breath with movement, it lowers heart rate and reduces muscle tension. This is the opposite of the “fight-or-flight” state that keeps people tossing and turning.

In a clinical trial at UCLA, older adults with insomnia who practiced tai chi three times a week reported significant improvements in both sleep quality and duration compared to a control group. The researchers noted that tai chi not only helped them fall asleep faster but also improved the depth of their rest.

Simple Tai Chi Wind-Down Practices

You do not need a full class to benefit. A few simple movements before bed can make a difference.

- **Floating Arms:** Stand with feet shoulder-width apart. Inhale as you

slowly raise your arms to chest height, exhale as you lower them. Repeat five times, moving with the breath.
- **Swaying Like Bamboo:** Shift weight gently from one foot to the other, letting the arms swing naturally at your sides. This calms the nervous system and releases tension in the lower back.
- **Gathering the Moon:** Circle the arms overhead as if scooping a ball of light, then lower them down the center of the body. Imagine drawing calm into yourself.

These movements are not strenuous, but their rhythm and imagery help quiet the mind.

Creating a Sleep-Friendly Routine

Pair tai chi practice with other simple habits: dim the lights an hour before bed, avoid screens, and keep the room slightly cool. Doing the same movements in the same order each night reinforces the signal to your brain that sleep is approaching.

One man in his late sixties described his routine this way: "I used to pace the living room worrying about the next day. Now I do ten minutes of tai chi, turn off the lights, and by the time my head hits the pillow, I'm already halfway to sleep."

Beyond Falling Asleep

The benefits extend into the night itself. Many practitioners report waking less often, and when they do, they fall back asleep more easily. This may be because tai chi reduces overall levels of arousal in the nervous system. With less background tension, the body is less likely to be jolted awake by small noises or discomforts.

Sleep problems are not solved by willpower alone—you cannot force yourself to relax. But you can create conditions that invite sleep, and tai chi provides a gentle, reliable method to do just that.

CHAPTER 4
ADAPTING FOR REAL BODIES

Seated & Supported Options (Chair, Counter, Wall)

Not every body moves the same way, and that's perfectly fine. Tai chi was never meant to be rigid—it adapts to the person, not the other way around. Chairs, counters, and walls can all be allies in practice, making movements accessible and safe while still delivering the same sense of calm, balance, and flow.

Seated Tai Chi: Moving Without Standing

Practicing from a chair is not second best—it's simply a different form. In fact, seated tai chi is widely used in rehabilitation clinics and senior centers because it allows you to focus on upper body flow and breath without worrying about balance.

A sturdy, armless chair works best. Sit with feet flat on the floor, knees at hip-width, and spine comfortably upright. From here, many classic tai chi moves translate beautifully. For example, "Parting the Horse's Mane" becomes a graceful forward-and-back arm movement, paired with subtle shifts in the torso. Breathing guides the rhythm, so the experience remains meditative.

In a study at the Mayo Clinic, participants who practiced seated tai chi for twelve weeks reported improvements in mood, energy, and pain management. One woman with arthritis in her knees described it as "a way to dance again without fear."

Using a Counter: Stability at Arm's Reach

Counters provide an ideal practice partner when you want the benefits of standing but prefer extra stability. Stand about half an arm's length away, feet hip-width apart, and place fingertips lightly on the surface. The key is to use the counter for reassurance, not as a crutch.

With this setup, you can practice shifting weight side to side or forward and back, gradually training the legs and hips. Movements like "Wave Hands Like Clouds" become accessible because you know the counter is there if you wobble. Over time, many practitioners notice they rely less on the counter, their confidence growing step by step.

Care homes often encourage this method because it allows residents to practice in familiar spaces, like kitchens or dining rooms, without needing specialized equipment.

The Wall: Support and Feedback

Walls offer a unique kind of help—they give both support and feedback. Standing with your back gently against the wall can remind you to keep posture upright, avoiding the common tendency to hunch forward.

The wall also works well for leg strengthening. For example, practicing a mini squat with the wall behind you builds thigh strength while removing fear of falling backward. Another option is standing side-on to the wall, sliding a hand lightly along its surface while stepping sideways. This keeps movements controlled yet fluid.

Tai chi instructors sometimes use the phrase "wall wisdom" to describe this method, because the wall quietly teaches alignment without saying a word.

Blending Seated and Supported Options

Support does not have to be all or nothing. Some days you may prefer to begin seated, then move to counter practice, and finally try a few steps without support. Other days, staying seated the entire time may feel right. The flexibility is part of the strength of tai chi—it meets you exactly where you are.

One veteran recovering from hip surgery described his approach: "I started with a chair for everything. Then I moved to the kitchen counter. Now, I only touch the counter at the start, just to check my balance. It's been like having training wheels I can remove when I'm ready."

Why Supported Tai Chi Works

Supportive practice does more than prevent falls. It reduces fear, and reducing fear unlocks the ability to move more freely. When the mind feels safe, the body relaxes, and movements become smoother. For seniors who may have experienced a fall in the past, this sense of safety is often the difference between avoiding activity and rediscovering joy in movement.

Whether you choose a chair, a counter, or a wall, the principle remains the same: tai chi is not about forcing the body into one mold. It is about creating flow, stability, and calm in whatever way works best for you.

Working with Arthritis, Back Pain or Joint Replacements

Bodies carry stories, and for many older adults, those stories include arthritis, aching backs, or even new hips and knees. These conditions can feel like barriers to activity, but tai chi is uniquely suited to work with—not against—them. Its slow, deliberate movements reduce strain, encourage circulation, and allow adjustments to fit each person's needs.

Arthritis: Moving Joints Without Aggravating Them

Arthritis often discourages people from moving, yet movement is exactly what joints need. The challenge is finding motion that keeps joints lubricated without overloading them. Tai chi fits the bill because it emphasizes gentle range-of-motion exercises and avoids sudden impact.

Take the knees, for example. Instead of bending deeply, tai chi teaches soft flexion, shifting weight gradually from one leg to the other. This nourishes the cartilage and strengthens surrounding muscles, easing pressure on the joint. A 2010 study published in *Arthritis Care & Research* found that seniors with knee osteoarthritis who practiced tai chi twice a week reported less pain and better function than those in a control group.

One woman with rheumatoid arthritis described tai chi as "the first exercise where I didn't have to pay for it with two days of pain."

Back Pain: Building Stability Through Gentle Motion

Chronic back pain is another common challenge. Many people tighten their core muscles instinctively to "protect" the spine, but over time this rigidity creates more pain. Tai chi counters this by promoting fluid, circular movements that engage the core without bracing.

Movements such as "Wave Hands Like Clouds" or gentle waist rotations encourage mobility in the spine while also strengthening the deep abdominal muscles. Controlled weight shifts build leg strength, which reduces the load carried by the lower back.

In clinical trials, tai chi has been shown to reduce disability in people with chronic low back pain. The mechanism is both physical and psychological: the movements increase strength and flexibility, while the mindful breathing reduces tension that can amplify pain.

One retired construction worker explained that after years of guarding his back, tai chi taught him to "move like water instead of like a plank."

Joint Replacements: Respecting New Limits While Regaining Confidence

Hip and knee replacements give many people a second chance at mobility, but they also come with fears. After surgery, it is common to feel cautious about putting weight on the new joint or moving in ways that might dislodge it. Tai chi's slow pace allows patients to rebuild trust in their bodies.

Standing exercises can begin with very small steps, using a counter or chair for stability. Gradually, as strength returns, steps become larger and more natural. Unlike some fitness routines, tai chi does not require kneeling, jumping, or twisting at speed—movements that might be risky for artificial joints.

Orthopedic surgeons often recommend low-impact activities after joint replacement, and tai chi fits that category perfectly. A 2019 review of rehabilitation studies noted that tai chi improved balance and reduced fear of falling among patients with hip replacements.

A veteran who had both knees replaced once said, "I was nervous about every step. Tai chi gave me the chance to relearn walking in a way that felt safe, almost like retraining my brain along with my legs."

Adapting Practice to the Body You Have

Every condition is different, so personalization matters. Some people may prefer shorter sessions—ten minutes instead of thirty. Others might need seated options for part of the routine. Pain is a guide here: mild discomfort as muscles stretch is normal, but sharp or worsening pain is a sign to adjust.

Helpful adaptations include:

- Keeping movements smaller and closer to the body.
- Using a chair, counter, or wall for balance support.
- Focusing more on upper body flow if legs feel unstable.
- Slowing down transitions between movements to reduce strain.

The Bigger Picture: Confidence and Quality of Life

Beyond the physical mechanics, tai chi offers something equally valuable—confidence. Arthritis, back pain, and joint replacements can all lead to fear of movement, which shrinks independence. By providing a safe way to move, tai chi breaks that cycle.

Research from Harvard Medical School emphasizes this point: participants not only improved physically but also reported greater enjoyment of daily life, from gardening to playing with grandchildren. When pain no longer dictates every choice, life feels larger again.

Working with arthritis, back pain, or joint replacements does not mean stepping aside from activity. It means moving with wisdom, adapting where necessary, and rediscovering what the body can do.

Precautions for Blood Pressure, Diabetes & Dizziness

Tai chi is often called "meditation in motion," but for people living with health conditions like blood pressure changes, diabetes, or dizziness, it's also a practice in safety. Gentle as it is, tai chi still shifts circulation, blood sugar, and balance. With a few smart precautions, you can enjoy all the benefits while avoiding the pitfalls.

Blood Pressure: Watching the Ups and Downs

High blood pressure is common in older adults, and while tai chi can help regulate it over time, sudden shifts in posture may temporarily affect readings. Moving too quickly from sitting to standing can cause lightheadedness, especially if you're on medication that dilates blood vessels.

One simple precaution is to rise gradually, giving your body time to adjust. When practicing tai chi, avoid locking the knees—keeping a gentle bend helps maintain steady circulation. Deep breathing is also helpful, as slow exhales activate the parasympathetic nervous system, which naturally lowers blood pressure.

For those with low blood pressure, the risk can be the opposite: dizziness from standing too long or from slow movements that reduce muscle pumping. In this case, shorter practice sessions or using a counter for stability can prevent faintness. Doctors often recommend checking blood pressure at home regularly, so pairing readings with your practice can provide reassurance.

Diabetes: Timing and Awareness

For people with diabetes, blood sugar can swing with activity. Tai chi is not as intense as jogging, but even moderate movement can lower glucose levels. Practicing on an empty stomach, especially if you've taken insulin or other medication, may increase the risk of hypoglycemia (low blood sugar).

A practical safeguard is to have a light snack before practice and keep glucose tablets or juice nearby, just in case. Many instructors encourage students with diabetes to check their sugar levels before and after sessions.

The benefits, however, are significant. Research has shown that tai chi improves insulin sensitivity and reduces stress hormones that can raise blood sugar. One long-term study in Shanghai found that older adults practicing tai chi regularly had better blood sugar control compared to those doing only walking exercises.

Neuropathy, a complication of diabetes, can dull sensation in the feet. This makes balance trickier, as the brain gets less information about the ground. Here, extra attention to foot placement is key, along with the use of stable shoes and, if needed, a supportive surface like a wall or rail.

Dizziness: Balancing the Inner Ear and Confidence

Dizziness may come from blood pressure changes, inner ear issues, or side effects of medication. It can be unsettling, especially for those already worried about falling. Tai chi is particularly valuable here because it trains the body to adjust balance through small, controlled shifts rather than abrupt motions.

Still, precautions help. If dizziness is frequent, practice near a sturdy support. Begin with smaller ranges of motion and build gradually. Some find that closing the eyes increases dizziness, so keeping the gaze steady at eye level can reduce symptoms.

Vestibular therapists sometimes recommend tai chi-like exercises to patients with inner ear disorders. The slow head turns and gentle weight shifts strengthen the brain's ability to recalibrate balance, making everyday movements—like turning to greet someone—less destabilizing.

Combining Precautions Without Losing Flow

It's easy to worry that all these precautions will make tai chi feel stiff or cautious, but in reality, they simply make the practice more personal. A man with high blood pressure may pause between postures to let his circulation adjust. A woman with diabetes may practice after a small snack and keep a chair nearby. Someone with dizziness may limit turning movements at first.

What matters is not perfection but consistency. The National Institutes of Health highlights tai chi as one of the safest activities for older adults, provided it's adapted to individual needs. The key is to listen to your body, respect its signals, and give yourself permission to modify movements when necessary.

The body may carry conditions like high blood pressure, diabetes, or dizziness, but with thoughtful adjustments, it can still experience the calm, flow, and balance that tai chi offers.

Progress Tracking: 4-Week Scorecard & Mini-Checks

One of the quiet frustrations in starting a new practice is not knowing whether it's "working." Tai chi doesn't give you quick wins like lifting heavier weights or running faster miles. Its progress is subtle: steadier steps, calmer breathing, fewer stumbles. That's why creating a simple scorecard and mini-checks can make the journey more visible and motivating.

Why Track Progress in Tai Chi?

Progress tracking isn't about competition—it's about awareness. By noticing small shifts in balance, posture, or confidence, you reinforce the value of showing up consistently. This is especially important for older adults who may be skeptical of whether such slow movements can actually change their bodies.

Researchers studying tai chi for seniors often use balance tests, walking speed, and self-reported quality of life to measure impact. You don't need a lab to do the same; you just need a simple system that captures how you're feeling and moving over time.

The 4-Week Scorecard

A four-week cycle provides enough time to notice changes without feeling overwhelming. Each week, you record how you're doing in a few key areas:

- **Balance:** Did you feel steadier when walking or standing?
- **Energy:** Did you have more or less stamina during daily activities?
- **Mood:** Did you feel calmer, less anxious, or better rested?
- **Mobility:** Were simple tasks like bending, reaching, or turning easier?
- **Confidence:** Did you feel less fearful of falling or moving?

You can rate each category on a scale of 1 to 5, with 1 being poor and 5 being excellent. At the end of four weeks, look at your ratings side by side. Often, even if balance feels the same, mood or confidence will show improvement. That matters just as much.

One senior I worked with initially gave herself low scores on balance but high ones on mood and sleep after four weeks. "I may still wobble, but I'm sleeping better than I have in years," she said. That was progress worth celebrating.

Mini-Checks for Everyday Feedback

In addition to the weekly scorecard, mini-checks keep you tuned in day by day. These are short, easy self-tests you can do at home.

- **Sit-to-Stand Test:** How many times can you rise from a chair without using your hands in 30 seconds? Note the number and track it over time.
- **Single-Leg Stand:** Stand near a counter and lift one foot an inch off the floor. How long can you balance without support?
- **Breath Check:** After a few minutes of tai chi, notice if your breathing feels deeper or calmer compared to before.
- **Mood Snapshot:** Rate your stress or calmness on a 1–10 scale before and

after practice.

These checks don't need to be formal. They're simply ways to notice change as it happens.

Making Tracking Enjoyable

The best progress systems are the ones you actually use. Some people prefer writing in a notebook, while others enjoy hanging a chart on the fridge. A few like using colored stickers—green for good days, yellow for okay, red for tough ones. The visual pattern itself can be motivating.

Tai chi groups sometimes share their progress at the end of class. One participant might say, "I can climb my stairs without pulling on the railing now," while another notes, "I don't feel as winded when I walk to the mailbox." These stories remind everyone that progress isn't always measured in numbers.

Building a Habit of Reflection

Progress tracking also trains mindfulness. By pausing to notice how you feel, you're reinforcing the very awareness that tai chi cultivates. Instead of waiting for a big breakthrough, you learn to appreciate steady, incremental change.

CHAPTER 5

ESSENTIAL STARTER SEQUENCE

Laying the Foundation with Gentle Movements

Starting any new practice is like planting seeds—you don't rush into it expecting a full-grown tree overnight. Instead, you give those seeds the right soil, water, and sunlight. Gentle movements act as that fertile ground for your body. They aren't meant to impress anyone or push your limits; they're here to help you build stability, awareness, and comfort so you can grow stronger step by step.

Why Gentle Matters First

Many people are tempted to skip the "easy" stuff. After all, if you've seen exercise videos online, the most dramatic routines usually involve speed, intensity, or complex steps. But here's the truth: the body, especially as it matures, doesn't thrive on shock or force—it thrives on consistency and safety. Starting with gentle movements allows your muscles, joints, and balance system to adapt gradually. Think of it as giving your nervous system a clear message: "We're moving, but we're moving safely."

In rehabilitation clinics, therapists often start patients recovering from surgery or injury with the simplest range-of-motion movements—raising arms, turning the neck, shifting weight side to side. Why? Because these actions retrain the body to feel stable, rebuild confidence, and prevent setbacks. The same principle applies here: your "starter sequence" isn't a warm-up for harder things; it is the heart of your training.

The Role of Balance and Posture

Gentle foundational exercises prioritize posture and balance above all else. When you stand with soft knees, or breathe while sweeping your arms, you're not just stretching—you're teaching your body to recognize its center. Balance is not something you lose overnight; it fades slowly if it isn't used. That's why many seniors notice they stumble more often, even if they feel strong otherwise. By practicing steady, grounded movements, you rebuild that hidden skill before it slips away further.

Consider the act of standing evenly on both feet. For most, it feels automatic. Yet research shows that weight is often unknowingly distributed unevenly—favoring one hip, locking one knee, or leaning slightly forward. Gentle practice shines a light on these small imbalances and helps correct them before they become patterns that strain joints or increase fall risk.

Breathing as a Foundation

Movement without breath is like trying to row a boat without water—it doesn't carry you anywhere. These starter exercises emphasize breath because it fuels both your muscles and your nervous system. Slow, intentional breathing calms stress hormones, supports circulation, and increases oxygen flow. When you pair breathing with soft, mindful gestures, it creates rhythm and flow, turning simple motions into whole-body practices.

For example, in "Anchor Breath Sweep," the timing of the inhale and exhale isn't just for relaxation; it teaches the body to move in harmony with breath. This connection reduces stiffness and helps your movements feel natural rather than forced.

Gentle Doesn't Mean Ineffective

There's a misconception that if something doesn't make you sweat or ache the next day, it isn't "real exercise." That idea has done more harm than good, especially for older adults who end up pushing too far and injuring themselves. Gentle exercises build what might be called "quiet strength." It's the kind of strength that shows up when you rise from a chair without wobbling, walk on uneven ground without fear, or reach overhead without discomfort.

A study on fall prevention programs for seniors showed that consistent, low-intensity exercises—focused on posture, breathing, and balance—reduced fall risk more than traditional strength training alone. The power lies in repetition and control, not intensity.

The Mental Foundation

Beyond physical benefits, gentle foundational movements play a psychological role. They lower the barrier of entry, making the practice approachable. If you've ever felt nervous about exercise—worried you'll "do it wrong" or "look silly"—starting here strips away that fear. The exercises are simple, safe, and forgiving, designed so you can succeed from day one.

There's also joy in mastering the basics. Like learning to play a musical instrument, you don't skip scales just because you want to play songs. Scales teach coordination, timing, and sensitivity. These movements are your scales: they train body awareness so that, later, you can move into more complex flows with confidence and ease.

Building Your Base Layer

Think of these exercises as the underpainting of a canvas. Every brushstroke you add later will be supported by this first layer. With each soft knee bend, each calm sweep of the arms, each mindful breath, you're laying bricks in a foundation that will support more dynamic practice down the line. Without this groundwork, the more advanced sequences risk feeling unstable or even unsafe. With it, everything feels connected, natural, and secure.

Standing Mountain with Soft Knees

Duration: 1–2 minutes
Repetitions: 1–2 times

Steps

- Stand with feet hip-width apart, toes facing forward.
- Soften knees with a gentle bend, not locked.
- Arms rest at sides, palms inward.
- Lift through the crown of the head, chin level.
- Inhale through the nose, exhale through the mouth, relaxing shoulders.
- Feel weight evenly spread across both feet.

Goal

This pose helps improve posture, strengthen legs and ankles, calm the breath, and create a steady sense of grounding and stability.

Safety tips: Keep knees slightly bent to avoid strain; use a wall or chair for support if needed.

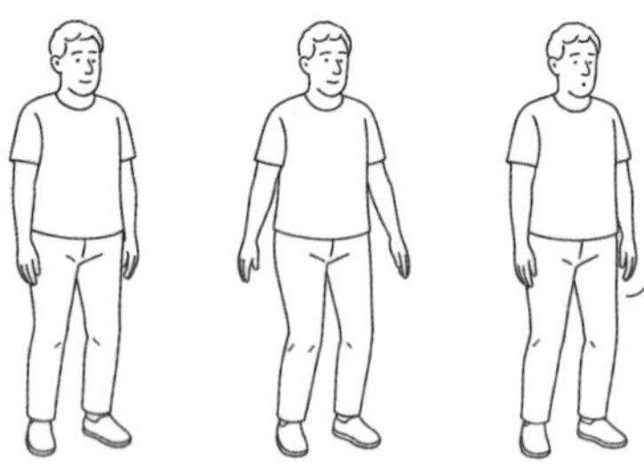

Anchor Breath Sweep

Duration: 1–2 minutes
Repetitions: 3–5 times

Steps

- Stand with feet hip-width apart, knees soft.
- Place hands lightly on the lower belly.
- Inhale slowly through the nose, letting the belly rise.
- Exhale as you sweep arms gently outward, palms facing down.
- Inhale again, guiding hands back toward the belly.
- Repeat with steady, flowing breath.

Goal

This pose supports calm breathing, eases tension in the chest, and connects breath with gentle arm movement for relaxation and focus.

Safety tips: Keep movements slow and avoid raising arms higher than comfortable.

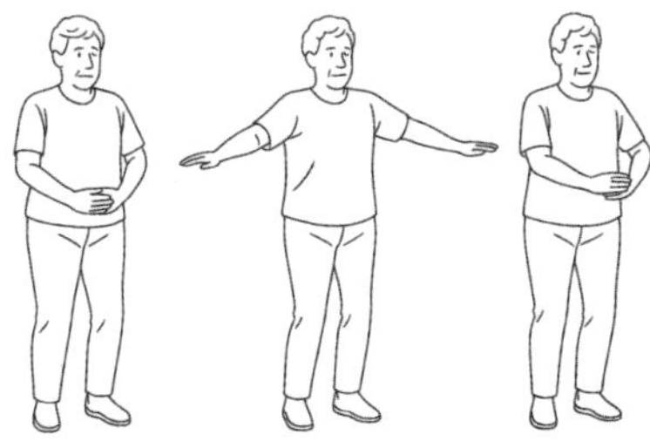

Floating Shoulder Clouds

Duration: 1–2 minutes
Repetitions: 4–6 times

Steps

- Stand with feet hip-width apart, knees relaxed.
- Inhale as you slowly lift shoulders toward the ears.
- Exhale as you roll shoulders back and down.
- Let arms and hands stay loose at the sides.
- Continue in smooth, cloudlike circles.

Goal

This pose loosens tight shoulders, improves circulation in the upper body, and encourages calm breathing to reduce stiffness.

Safety tips: Keep circles small if shoulder mobility is limited; stop if sharp pain occurs.

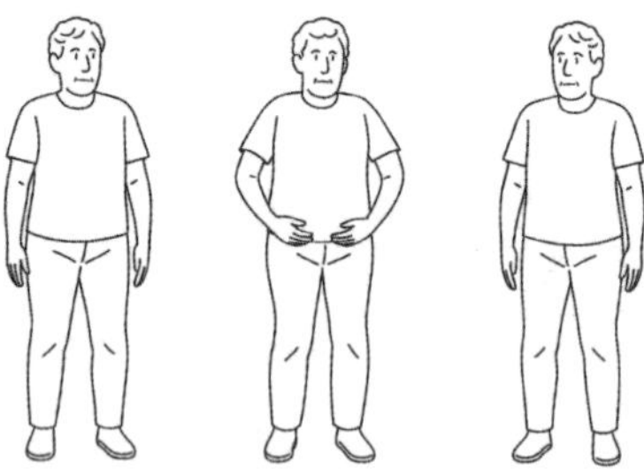

Gentle Weight Shift (Knee-Friendly)

Duration: 1–2 minutes
Repetitions: 6–8 shifts

Steps

- Stand with feet slightly wider than hips, knees soft.
- Shift weight gently to the right foot, keeping knees relaxed.
- Return slowly to center.
- Shift weight to the left foot with the same ease.
- Continue side to side, moving slowly and smoothly.

Goal

This pose builds balance, strengthens legs without stress on the knees, and improves awareness of weight distribution.

Safety tips: Hold a chair or counter nearby for support; keep steps small to avoid knee strain.

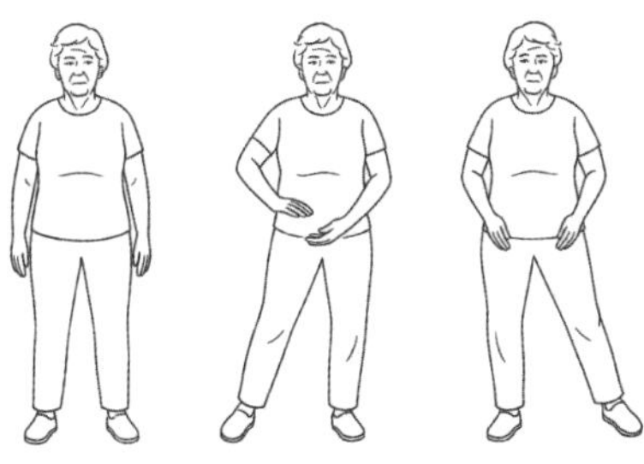

Open Gate Chest Fan

Duration: 1–2 minutes
Repetitions: 4–6 times

Steps

- Stand with feet hip-width apart, knees slightly bent.
- Bring palms together at chest level.
- Inhale as you slowly open arms outward, like opening a gate.
- Exhale as you bring palms gently back together.
- Keep shoulders relaxed and movements smooth.

Goal

This pose expands the chest, improves breathing capacity, and releases tightness in the upper body while promoting calm focus.

Safety tips: Avoid overstretching arms; move within a comfortable range.

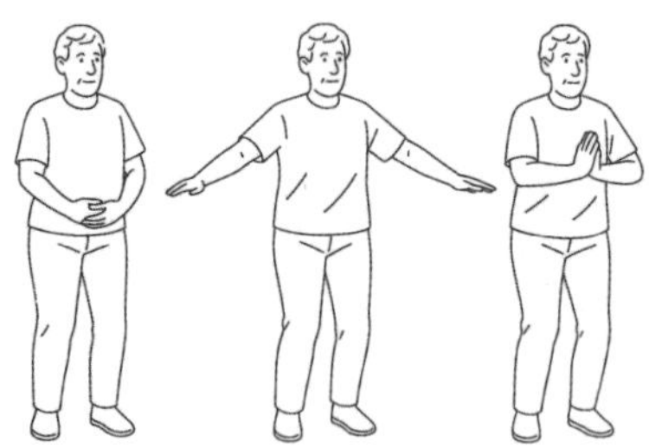

River Hands Forward Flow

Duration: 1–2 minutes
Repetitions: 4–6 times

Steps

- Stand with feet shoulder-width apart, knees soft.
- Rest hands near the waist, palms facing down.
- Inhale as you slowly move arms forward, palms gliding like water.
- Exhale as you draw hands gently back toward the body.
- Repeat with smooth, flowing rhythm.

Goal

This pose calms the mind, supports shoulder mobility, and connects breath with gentle flowing movement for relaxation.

Safety tips: Keep arm movements low and easy; avoid locking elbows.

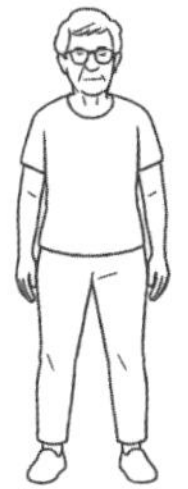
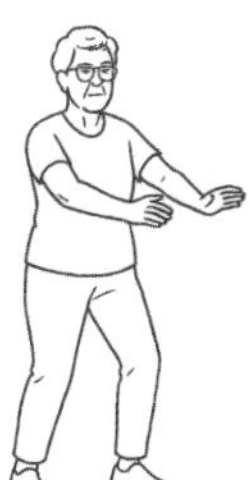
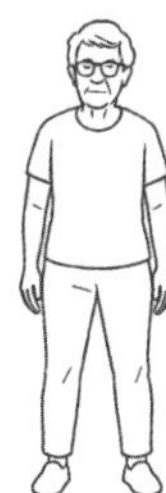

Pebble Heel Tap

Duration: 1–2 minutes
Repetitions: 6–8 taps per foot

Steps

- Stand with feet hip-width apart, knees relaxed.
- Shift weight slightly onto the left foot.
- Extend right foot forward and tap the heel lightly on the floor.
- Return foot to starting position.
- Repeat on the opposite side, alternating feet.

Goal

This pose strengthens ankles, improves coordination, and builds gentle stability for walking and balance.

Safety tips: Hold onto a chair or counter if balance feels unsteady; keep taps light and controlled.

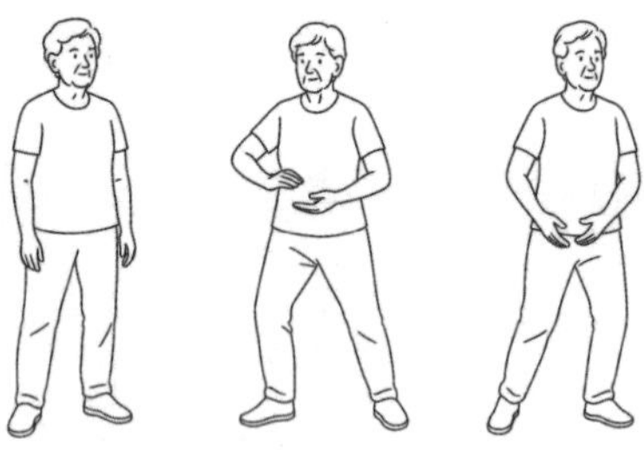

CHAPTER 6

WEEK 1 — BUILD YOUR BASE: CONFIDENCE & STABILITY

Building Balance and Confidence Step by Step

Balance is one of those things you don't think about until it slips away. Maybe it's a stumble on an uneven sidewalk, or the nervousness you feel stepping off a bus. These moments aren't just about muscle strength; they're about trust—trust in your body to support you when you need it most. Rebuilding that trust doesn't happen in a single leap. It happens step by step, in small, steady practices that remind your body how to stay upright, how to move with control, and how to feel safe doing so.

Balance as a Learned Skill

Balance isn't something you either have or don't have. It's a skill that can be trained and retrained. In fact, physical therapists often describe it as a "use it or lose it" ability. As people age, balance tends to decline not because the body has given up, but because daily life no longer challenges it. Think about it: most of us walk on flat floors, sit in supportive chairs, and rarely bend, twist, or shift weight outside of familiar patterns. Without variety, the body forgets. By practicing gentle, structured steps, you reintroduce your system to the micro-adjustments it once handled automatically.

Confidence Through Movement

Confidence grows from experience. If you've ever hesitated before stepping off a curb, it's not only your muscles that pause—it's your mind remembering past slips or fearing the next one. Gentle, repeatable exercises serve as safe experiments. Each time you shift weight, sway, or rock side to side without falling, you prove to yourself that your body is capable. That repeated proof is what rebuilds confidence. And confidence, in turn, encourages more movement in daily life—walking to the park, dancing at a wedding, or simply reaching for something on a high shelf without hesitation.

The Role of Small Steps

Some might wonder, "Why such small, simple movements?" The answer is that small steps lay the groundwork for bigger ones. Imagine building a bridge: you don't begin with the arch; you start with supports. Exercises like side-to-side rocking or gentle arm sweeps strengthen the "supports" of balance—ankle stability, core control, and coordination between breath and movement. Once those are steady, the body naturally handles more complex actions.

A Practical Example

Consider the "Side-to-Side Rocking Step" you'll practice in this week's sequence. On the surface, it looks like swaying your weight back and forth. But underneath, several things are happening: your ankles are adjusting to shifts, your knees are learning to soften instead of lock, your hips are guiding balance, and your core is keeping everything aligned. Practicing this repeatedly helps retrain these systems to work together. It's the same skill you need when you're stepping out of a car, walking on grass, or turning quickly when someone calls your name.

The Breath-Balance Connection

Confidence isn't only physical—it's also mental. Breath is a quiet but powerful partner in this. Shallow, anxious breathing often appears when someone feels unstable. By pairing steady breathing with balance exercises, you train your nervous system to stay calm even as the body shifts. This reduces the fear of falling and encourages a sense of control. For example, in "Sunrise Heart Lift," the rising arms are timed with an inhale, teaching the body to expand upward with breath, while the exhale grounds you again.

Why Stability Before Strength

It's tempting to skip ahead to strengthening exercises—lifting weights, pushing resistance bands, or holding deep squats. But for many, those activities feel intimidating without a stable base. Building stability first is like making sure the floor is solid before moving furniture into the room. Stability gives strength a place to stand. That's why this week focuses less on resistance and more on control, posture, and slow, confident movement.

The Bigger Picture

Rebuilding balance and confidence is not about avoiding falls alone. It's about reclaiming independence. Every step you take without fear expands what you can do. It might be walking down stairs without gripping the rail so tightly, or standing tall in a crowd without worrying about being bumped. These aren't dramatic changes, but they shape the quality of daily life in profound ways. By focusing on simple, repeatable steps now, you set yourself up not just for safer movement, but for freer, more confident living.

Sunrise Heart Lift

Duration: 1–2 minutes
Repetitions: 3–5 times

Steps

- Stand with feet hip-width apart, knees soft.
- Place hands together at chest level.
- Inhale as you slowly lift arms upward, opening the chest.
- Exhale as you lower arms gently back down.
- Keep movements smooth and shoulders relaxed.

Goal

This pose opens the chest, encourages deep breathing, improves posture, and promotes calm energy.

Safety tips: Avoid raising arms higher than comfortable; keep movements slow and easy.

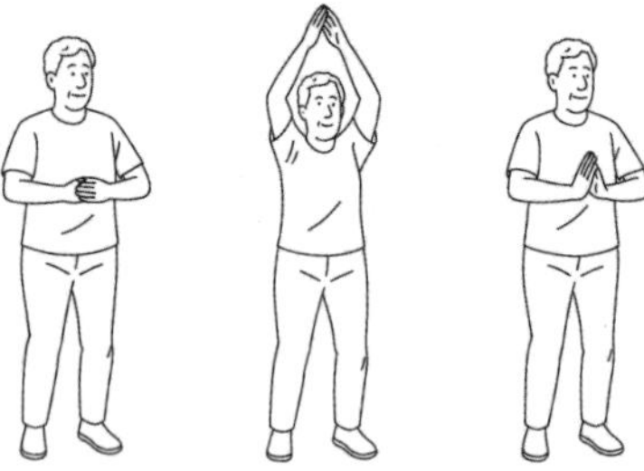

Side-to-Side Rocking Step

Duration: 1–2 minutes
Repetitions: 6–8 shifts

Steps

- Stand with feet wider than hips, knees slightly bent.
- Shift weight slowly to the right foot.
- Bring weight back to center.
- Shift weight gently to the left foot.
- Continue rocking side to side with steady rhythm.

Goal

This pose strengthens legs, trains balance, and increases awareness of weight transfer for safer movement.

Safety tips: Keep a chair nearby for support; avoid shifting too far if balance feels unsteady.

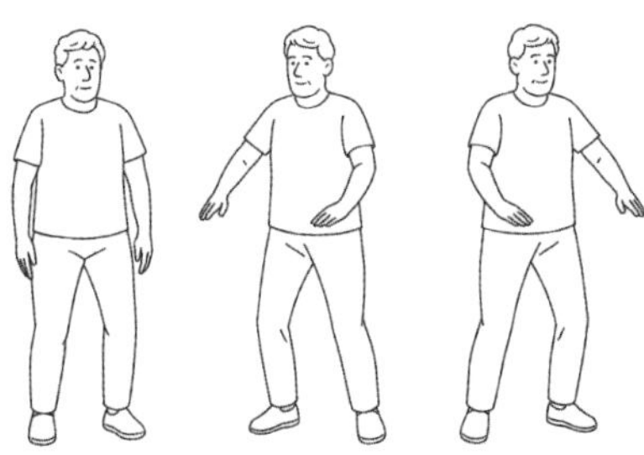

Turtle Neck Unwind

Duration: 1–2 minutes
Repetitions: 4–6 circles

Steps

- Sit or stand with feet flat and spine tall.
- Slowly drop chin toward chest.
- Gently roll head to the right, then back, then to the left.
- Keep movements small and relaxed.
- Repeat in the opposite direction.

Goal

This pose eases neck tension, improves flexibility, and relaxes shoulders for better posture.

Safety tips: Keep circles small to avoid strain; stop if dizziness occurs.

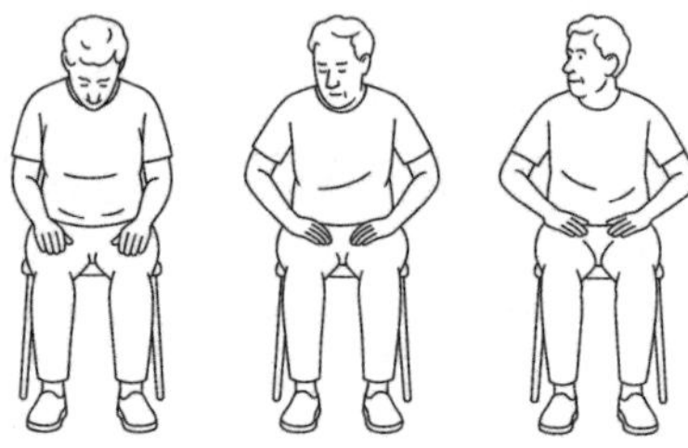

Lantern Raise & Lower

Duration: 1–2 minutes
Repetitions: 4–6 times

Steps

- Stand with feet shoulder-width apart, knees soft.
- Hold hands in front of the belly as if carrying a lantern.
- Inhale as you lift hands slowly to chest height.
- Exhale as you lower hands gently back down.
- Keep shoulders loose and breath steady.

Goal

This pose builds arm strength, connects breath with movement, and encourages relaxation.

Safety tips: Lift arms only to a comfortable height; avoid locking elbows.

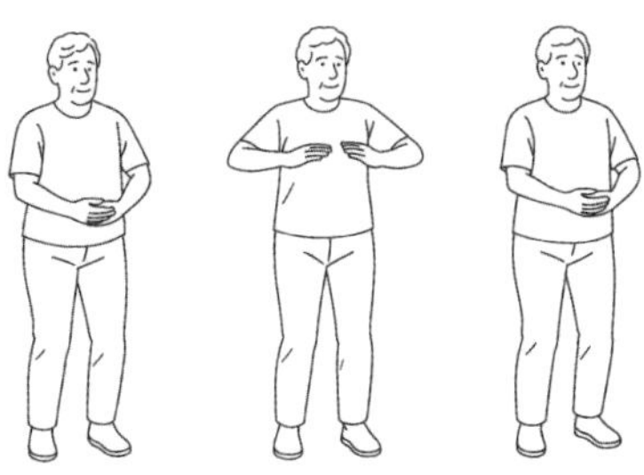

Willow Waist Turn

Duration: 1–2 minutes
Repetitions: 6–8 turns

Steps

- Stand with feet hip-width apart, knees slightly bent.
- Place hands loosely at the waist or let them swing naturally.
- Gently turn torso to the right.
- Return to center, then turn slowly to the left.
- Move side to side in a smooth rhythm.

Goal

This pose loosens the waist and spine, supports mobility, and improves circulation through gentle twisting.

Safety tips: Keep movements small and controlled; avoid forcing the twist.

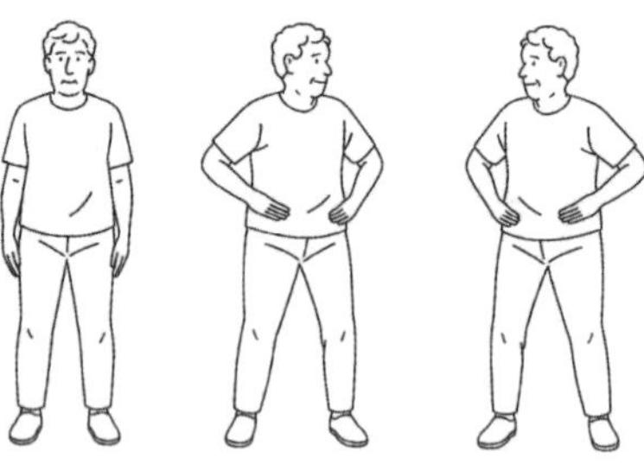

Skimming Water Arms

Duration: 1–2 minutes
Repetitions: 4–6 sweeps

Steps

- Stand with feet hip-width apart, knees relaxed.
- Extend arms slightly forward, palms facing down.
- Inhale as you sweep arms outward in a gentle arc.
- Exhale as arms return toward the body.
- Move hands as if gliding over water.

Goal

This pose promotes relaxation, improves shoulder mobility, and creates a flowing, calming rhythm.

Safety tips: Keep arm movements low; adjust range if shoulders feel tight.

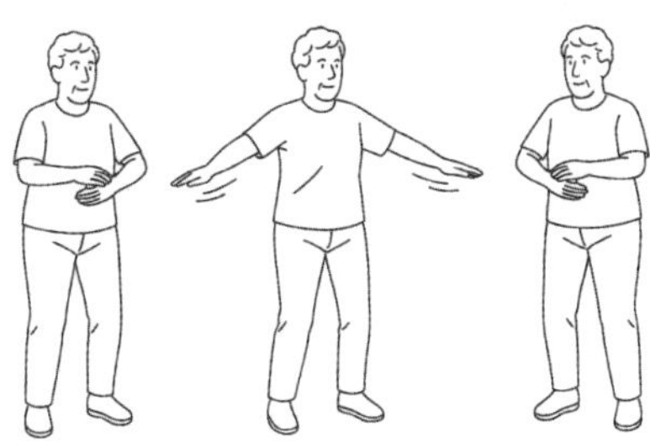

Palm Glide Across the Pond

Duration: 1–2 minutes
Repetitions: 6–8 glides

Steps

- Stand with feet hip-width apart, knees soft.
- Place palms in front of the body at waist level.
- Shift weight gently to the right foot as right palm glides outward.
- Return to center and repeat with left palm and foot.
- Continue alternating sides in a smooth rhythm.

Goal

This pose supports coordination, balance, and gentle strengthening of legs and arms while encouraging calm focus.

Safety tips: Keep steps small; use a chair or wall nearby if balance feels uncertain.

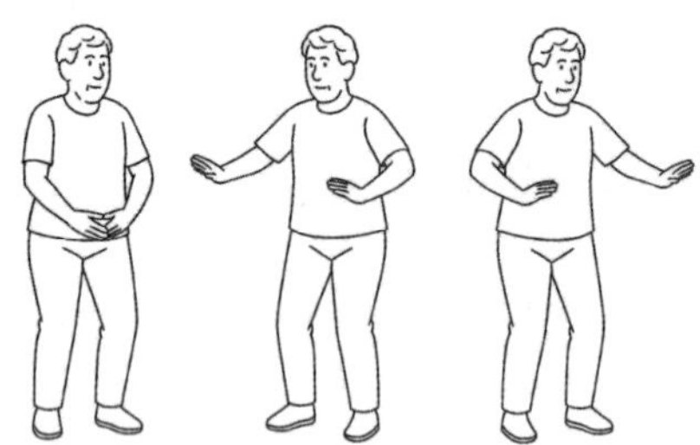

CHAPTER 7

WEEK 2 — SMOOTH FLOW: LIGHTNESS & MOBILITY

Flowing with Ease and Lightness

Movement doesn't have to feel heavy or mechanical. When the body finds rhythm and softness, it feels almost like water running downstream—steady, smooth, and unstoppable. This week's focus is on teaching your body to let go of stiffness and discover flow. Instead of fighting gravity or forcing motion, you'll practice moving with it, creating a sense of ease that not only helps mobility but also refreshes the mind.

Why Flow Matters

Many people associate exercise with effort—sweat, strain, and pushing through discomfort. While that may have its place, for older adults the goal is different: to restore lightness, to move without fear, and to feel comfortable in your own skin. Flow-based exercises teach your body to move in continuous patterns, so one action blends into the next. This has practical value. Think about walking across a room: it isn't a series of stops and starts; it's a smooth chain of steps. Training in flow mirrors how life actually moves.

The nervous system also benefits from fluid movement. Studies on Tai Chi show that flowing sequences reduce the "startle response" in older adults—the tendency to stiffen up when surprised. By practicing transitions, your body learns to adapt instead of freeze, lowering the risk of falls.

Releasing Stiffness

Lightness often comes when stiffness leaves. Stiffness might show up in the shoulders, the lower back, or the ankles. Exercises like the "Meadow

Shoulder Sweep" or "Windmill Wrist Spiral" aren't just gentle stretches—they are reminders to let joints move in circles, arcs, and waves. When you loosen these areas, you're not only increasing range of motion but also rediscovering the joy of easy movement.

Think of a rusted hinge: at first it creaks, but with steady oiling, it swings freely again. Your joints are no different. Practicing light spirals, reaches, and glides is the oil.

The Feeling of Lightness

Lightness isn't about body weight—it's about sensation. When you do the "Feather Heel Hover," for instance, the focus is on letting the foot feel as if it floats, rather than stamping down. This gentle hover sends a message to your brain: movement can be graceful, not clumsy. With repetition, everyday steps start to feel less heavy, more agile.

This is especially helpful for those who've noticed their gait becoming slower or more deliberate with age. By training in "light" movements, you're giving yourself the ability to walk more smoothly, making outings feel less like a chore and more like freedom.

Flow and Breath Together

You'll notice that many of these movements link directly to breathing. "Diagonal Hand Trail" connects inhaling with an upward reach and exhaling with a return to center. This pairing isn't random. When you sync breath and motion, you create rhythm. Rhythm is what makes flow possible. Without it, movements are just disconnected steps. With it, they become a dance.

This connection also supports relaxation. Shallow or erratic breathing tends to make the body tense. Deep, steady breathing signals calm, which allows muscles to soften. The softer the muscles, the lighter the movement.

Building Mobility Safely

Mobility is different from flexibility. Flexibility is about stretching further;

mobility is about using that stretch in real actions. For example, raising your arm overhead is flexibility. Raising it overhead while stepping forward with control is mobility. The exercises in this chapter focus on mobility because it's more practical for daily life.

Simple tasks like reaching into a cupboard, putting on a jacket, or bending slightly to tie a shoe all require mobility. Flow-based drills like the "Crescent Reach and Step" mimic these motions in a safe, low-intensity way, training you for the movements you'll actually use.

The Emotional Side of Flow

There's also an emotional benefit to feeling light. Flowing sequences encourage a mindset of ease rather than tension. People often report feeling not just physically refreshed but mentally uplifted after practicing flowing patterns. It's as if moving smoothly clears out some of the heaviness of stress.

Even the names of the exercises—"Meadow Shoulder Sweep," "Feather Heel Hover"—are chosen to evoke imagery of calm and nature. These associations matter. They give you something pleasant to focus on while moving, which makes the practice more enjoyable and more likely to become part of your daily routine.

Diagonal Hand Trail

Duration: 1–2 minutes
Repetitions: 4–6 times each side

Steps

- Stand with feet shoulder-width apart, knees soft.
- Place hands near the waist, palms facing inward.
- Inhale as you slowly extend the right hand diagonally upward.
- Exhale as you bring the hand back down to the waist.
- Repeat on the left side, alternating smoothly.

Goal

This pose improves coordination, opens the chest, strengthens the arms, and encourages graceful, flowing movement.

Safety tips: Avoid overstretching the arms; move only as far as is comfortable.

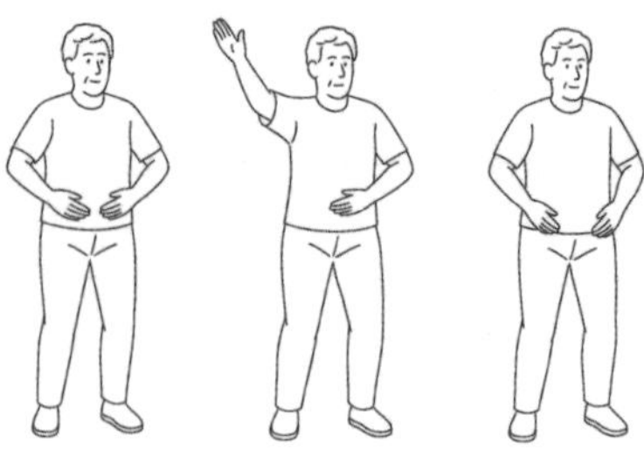

Crescent Reach and Step

Duration: 1–2 minutes
Repetitions: 4–6 steps each side

Steps

- Stand with feet hip-width apart, knees slightly bent.
- Step the right foot gently forward, keeping balance steady.
- Raise both arms in a soft crescent shape overhead.
- Exhale as you lower arms and step back to starting position.
- Repeat with the left foot, alternating sides.

Goal

This pose enhances balance, strengthens legs, and stretches the upper body while promoting lightness in movement.

Safety tips: Keep steps small; hold a chair or wall nearby if needed for balance.

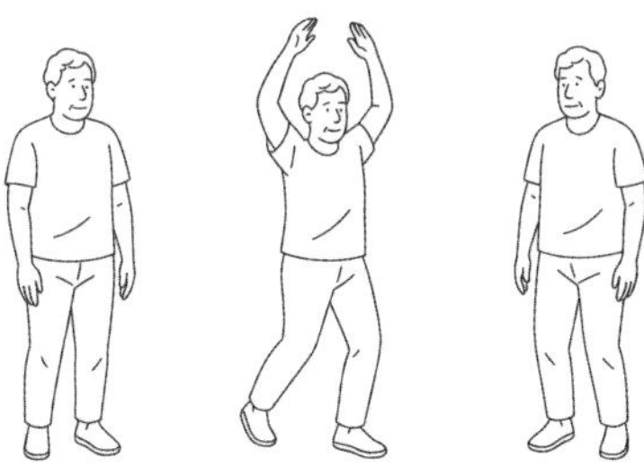

Windmill Wrist Spiral

Duration: 1–2 minutes
Repetitions: 6–8 spirals

Steps

- Stand with feet hip-width apart, knees relaxed.
- Lift arms slightly in front of the body, elbows soft.
- Rotate wrists slowly in outward circles, as if drawing spirals in the air.
- Continue spiraling smoothly, then reverse direction.
- Keep shoulders loose and breathing steady.

Goal

This pose loosens wrists, improves circulation in the hands, and builds mobility in the arms while calming the mind.

Safety tips: Keep wrist circles gentle; stop if any discomfort occurs.

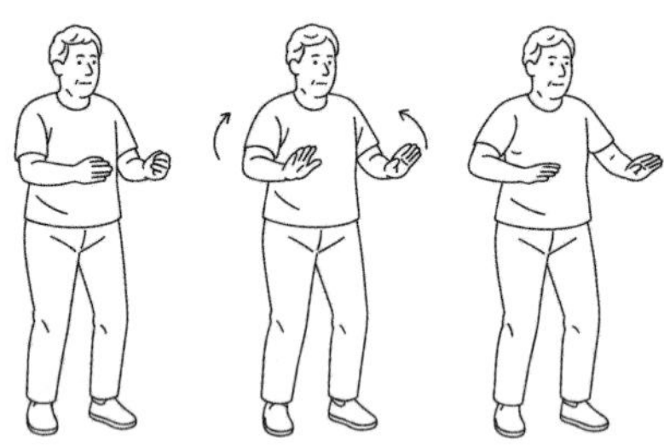

Feather Heel Hover

Duration: 1–2 minutes
Repetitions: 6–8 hovers per foot

Steps

- Stand tall with feet hip-width apart, knees soft.
- Shift weight gently to the left foot.
- Lift the right heel slightly off the floor, toes still touching.
- Lower the heel softly back down.
- Repeat on the other side, alternating slowly.

Goal

This pose strengthens ankles, improves stability, and trains gentle balance without strain on the knees.

Safety tips: Hold onto a wall or chair for support; keep lifts small and controlled.

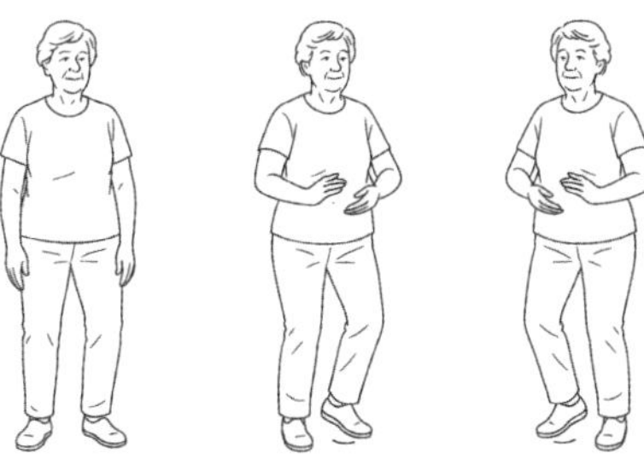

Gentle Archer Draw

Duration: 1–2 minutes
Repetitions: 4–6 draws each side

Steps

- Stand with feet wider than hips, knees slightly bent.
- Extend the left arm forward at shoulder height.
- Draw the right hand back as if pulling a bowstring.
- Exhale as you release the imaginary bowstring.
- Switch sides and repeat smoothly.

Goal

This pose builds coordination, strengthens the upper body, and encourages focus through mindful, deliberate movement.

Safety tips: Keep knees soft; do not overextend the shoulders.

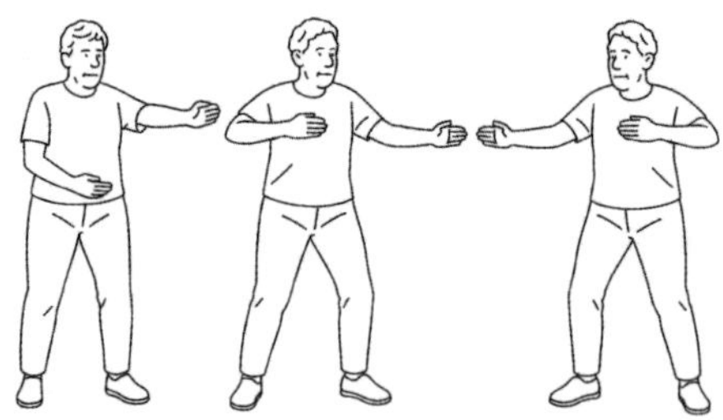

Drifting Hands Crossing

Duration: 1–2 minutes
Repetitions: 6–8 crossings

Steps

- Stand with feet shoulder-width apart, knees relaxed.
- Lift both arms in front of the chest, palms facing down.
- Cross the hands gently over each other.
- Open arms outward again with soft inhale.
- Repeat the crossing and opening in smooth rhythm.

Goal

This pose improves coordination, relaxes the shoulders, and supports a sense of flowing calm.

Safety tips: Keep movements gentle; avoid raising arms higher than comfortable.

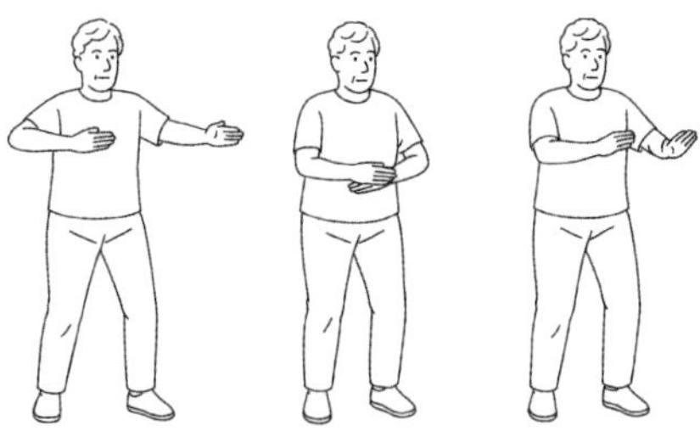

Meadow Shoulder Sweep

Duration: 1–2 minutes
Repetitions: 6–8 sweeps

Steps

- Stand with feet hip-width apart, knees soft.
- Let arms hang loosely at the sides.
- Sweep the right arm gently across the body at waist height.
- Return it slowly to the side.
- Repeat with the left arm, alternating in a gentle flow.

Goal

This pose releases shoulder stiffness, promotes smooth upper-body movement, and calms the breath.

Safety tips: Keep sweeps low and relaxed; avoid forcing shoulder movement.

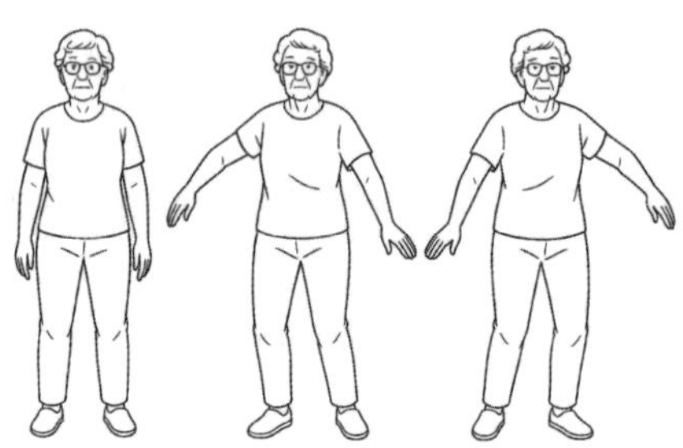

CHAPTER 8

WEEK 3 — GENTLE STRENGTH & COORDINATION

Strengthening the Body through Gentle Coordination

Strength isn't just about how much weight you can lift or how far you can stretch—it's about how well your body parts work together. Coordination is the glue that links strength with balance and stability. Without it, even simple tasks like stepping sideways or reaching overhead can feel awkward or unsafe. This chapter focuses on exercises that don't just build muscle in isolation but encourage the arms, legs, and core to move as a team. Think of it as teaching your body to play in harmony rather than as separate instruments.

Gentle Strength, Real Results

Some people imagine strength training as lifting heavy dumbbells or grinding through long repetitions at the gym. But research shows that for older adults, functional strength—the kind you use in everyday life—comes more from controlled bodyweight exercises and balance work than from traditional gym routines. A "gentle squat," for instance, may not look dramatic, but it builds the same muscles you rely on when rising from a chair or climbing stairs.

That's why these sequences avoid strain while still targeting key areas: legs for support, the core for stability, and arms for coordinated movement. Gentle strength is not less valuable; it's simply more practical and sustainable.

The Role of Coordination

Strength without coordination can lead to clumsy movement. Imagine trying to catch yourself after a stumble. Strong legs alone won't help if your arms don't react quickly, or if your core doesn't stabilize your torso. Coordination brings all these elements together.

Exercises like "Push the Moon" or "Crane Beak Touch" train the arms and breath to move in sync, while "Garden Gate Step" connects footwork with flowing upper-body gestures. Each repetition helps your body practice timing —an underrated but vital part of preventing falls and staying agile.

Everyday Examples

The link between strength and coordination shows up constantly in daily activities. Carrying groceries requires both arm strength and balance as you walk. Turning to place a dish on a high shelf requires core stability and shoulder mobility. Even brushing snow off a car demands coordinated twisting, reaching, and stepping. By practicing gentle but deliberate sequences, you prepare your body for these real-life scenarios.

Breathing as Part of Strength

Breath may not seem like a strength-builder, but it plays a major role in coordination. When you inhale during an upward reach or exhale during a lowering movement, you're teaching your body to use breath as a stabilizer. For example, in "Beltline Core Wrap," the circling motion is paired with steady breathing to gently activate abdominal muscles. This subtle training helps protect your spine and improves posture over time.

Why Gentle Still Builds Strength

Skeptics might argue that "gentle" can't build strength. Yet studies on older adults practicing Tai Chi or light resistance exercises show measurable improvements in muscle function, balance, and even bone density. The key is consistency, not intensity. Performing controlled squats, coordinated arm movements, and rhythmic steps several times a week adds up to real changes.

The advantage of gentle strength-building is safety. You're less likely to overwork joints, aggravate arthritis, or strain muscles. Instead of a cycle of "work hard, then recover from pain," you get steady, sustainable progress.

The Confidence Factor

Coordination isn't just physical—it also builds confidence. When your movements feel smooth and controlled, you trust your body more. That trust reduces hesitation, whether it's stepping off a bus, walking across wet grass, or trying a new dance step at a family gathering. Confidence turns strength into freedom: the freedom to move without second-guessing yourself.

Building the Foundation for the Future

These exercises aren't meant to be the finish line. They're part of a process that gradually equips your body to handle more. By mastering coordination now, you make later movements—whether it's a new flow sequence, a brisk walk, or even playing with grandchildren—more accessible and safe. The body, at any age, thrives on this kind of progressive challenge, especially when strength and coordination grow hand in hand.

Crane Beak Touch

Duration: 1–2 minutes
Repetitions: 4–6 times

Steps

- Stand with feet hip-width apart, knees soft.
- Bring fingertips together in front of the chest like a crane's beak.
- Inhale as you gently raise hands upward to eye level.
- Exhale as you lower hands slowly back down.
- Keep shoulders relaxed and movement steady.

Goal

This pose strengthens arms and shoulders, supports focus, and builds coordination through controlled hand movement.

Safety tips: Avoid lifting arms higher than comfortable; keep wrists relaxed.

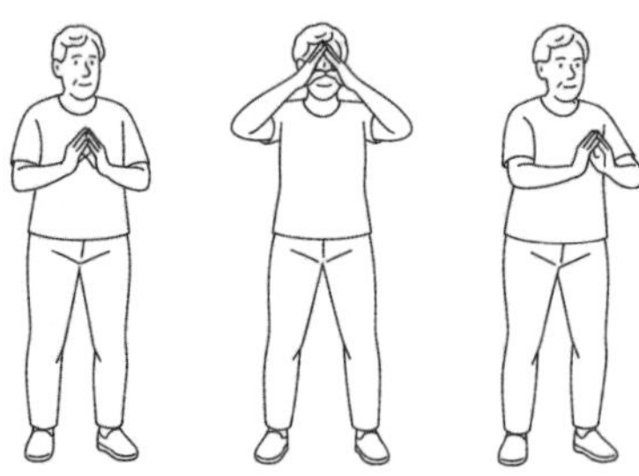

Beltline Core Wrap

Duration: 1–2 minutes
Repetitions: 6–8 wraps

Steps

- Stand with feet shoulder-width apart, knees relaxed.
- Place palms near the waistline.
- Circle hands gently around the beltline as if wrapping the core.
- Exhale as hands come forward, inhale as they circle back.
- Keep movements small and connected to the breath.

Goal

This pose engages the core, improves waist mobility, and supports gentle abdominal strength with relaxed breathing.

Safety tips: Keep circles soft; avoid twisting too far at the waist.

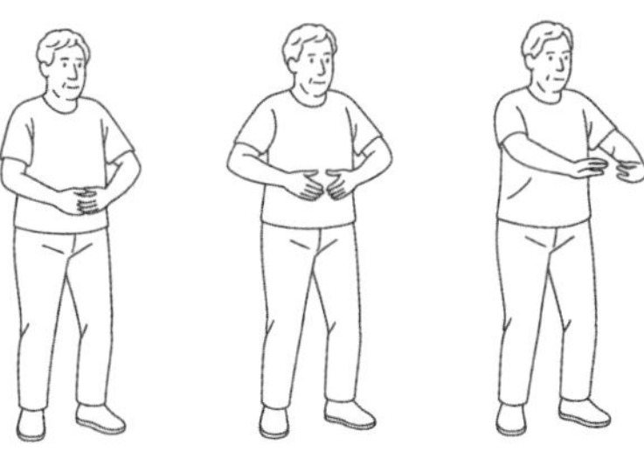

Riverside Side Stretch

Duration: 1–2 minutes
Repetitions: 3–4 stretches per side

Steps

- Stand tall with feet hip-width apart, knees soft.
- Place right hand on the hip for support.
- Inhale as you raise the left arm overhead.
- Exhale as you gently lean to the right side.
- Return slowly to center and switch sides.

Goal

This pose stretches the sides of the body, improves flexibility in the waist, and supports relaxed breathing.

Safety tips: Keep the lean gentle; avoid bending too far or locking the knees.

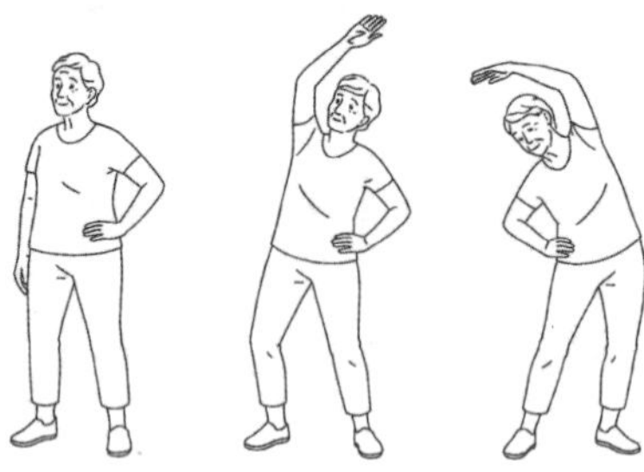

Push the Moon

Duration: 1–2 minutes
Repetitions: 4–6 presses

Steps

- Stand with feet hip-width apart, knees slightly bent.
- Hold palms together at chest height.
- Inhale as you press palms forward slowly.
- Exhale as you draw palms gently back toward the chest.
- Repeat with steady rhythm, arms relaxed.

Goal

This pose strengthens arms and chest, supports coordination, and encourages calm, rhythmic breathing.

Safety tips: Keep elbows soft; avoid pushing arms too far forward.

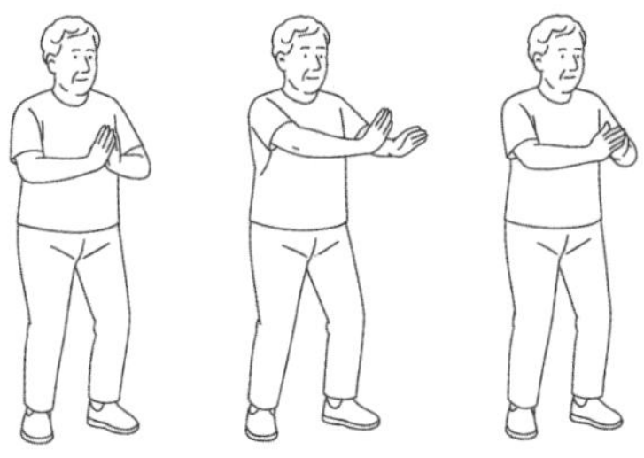

Garden Gate Step

Duration: 1–2 minutes
Repetitions: 4–6 steps each side

Steps

- Stand tall with feet together, knees relaxed.
- Step the right foot gently to the side.
- Inhale as you open both arms outward like a gate.
- Exhale as you step back to center, arms returning inward.
- Repeat on the left side, alternating smoothly.

Goal

This pose improves balance, strengthens legs, and supports coordination with flowing arm and leg movement.

Safety tips: Keep steps small; hold a chair nearby if extra support is needed.

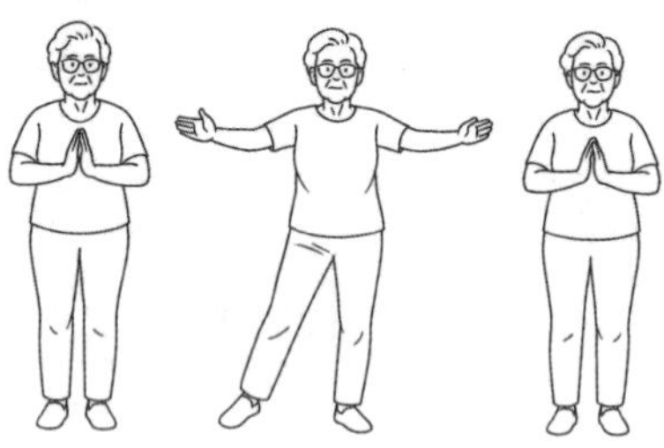

Brush Heel & Lift

Duration: 1–2 minutes
Repetitions: 4–6 lifts per foot

Steps

- Stand with feet shoulder-width apart, knees soft.
- Shift weight gently onto the left foot.
- Brush right heel lightly forward along the floor.
- Lift the heel a few inches, keeping toes touching.
- Return foot to starting position and switch sides.

Goal

This pose strengthens ankles and legs, improves coordination, and encourages balance through gentle controlled lifts.

Safety tips: Keep lifts low; use a chair or wall for support if needed.

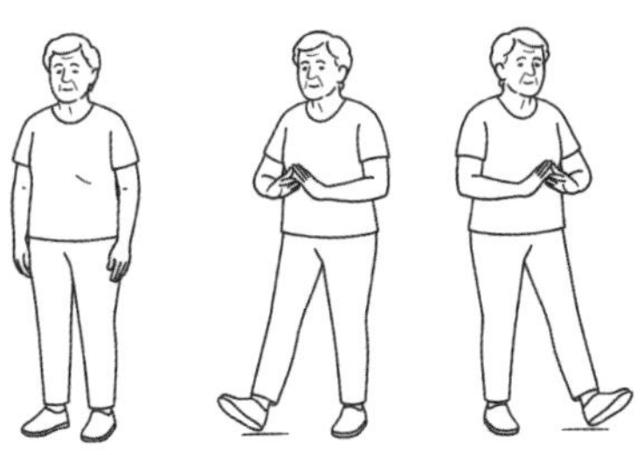

Bamboo Kneel-Free Squat

Duration: 1–2 minutes
Repetitions: 6–8 squats

Steps

- Stand with feet wider than hips, toes pointing forward.
- Bend knees slightly as if lowering into a soft squat.
- Keep back straight and chest lifted.
- Inhale as you rise slowly back to standing.
- Exhale as you bend gently again, keeping movement light.

Goal

This pose strengthens legs, supports joint stability, and builds coordination without putting pressure on the knees.

Safety tips: Keep squats shallow; hold a chair or counter for support if balance is unsteady.

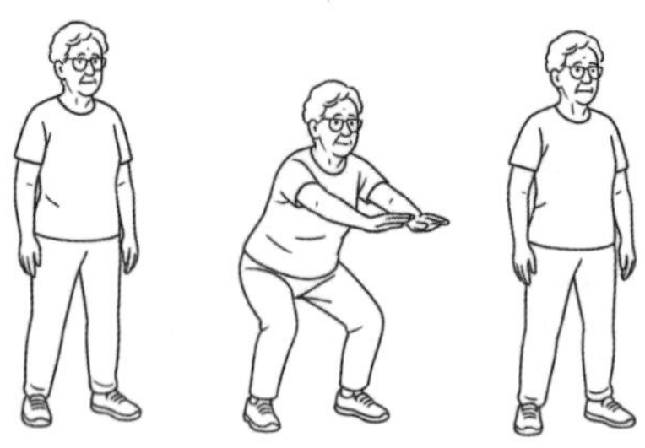

CHAPTER 9

WEEK 4 — INTEGRATION: BODY, BREATH & BALANCE

Uniting Breath, Body, and Balance into Harmony

Harmony isn't something abstract; it's something you feel when every part of you is working together. Breath, body, and balance are like three strands of rope—individually they can fray, but twisted together they become strong and reliable. This week focuses on weaving those strands into daily movement so that strength doesn't stand apart from calm, and balance doesn't happen without breath.

The Role of Breath in Movement

Breath is often treated as separate from exercise, but it is the silent driver of stability and calm. When you inhale deeply, your ribcage expands, your spine lengthens slightly, and your nervous system receives a signal of safety. Exhaling does more than release air—it softens tension and helps your muscles ground into the floor.

Consider how you feel when startled. The breath catches, muscles tighten, and balance is compromised. Now imagine pairing each shift of weight or lift of the arms with deliberate breathing. Suddenly the movement feels steadier, less reactive. That's why in practices like Tai Chi or Qigong, every gesture is timed to inhale or exhale—it teaches the body to stay calm even in transition.

Balance as More Than Standing Still

People often assume balance means holding a static pose. In reality, balance is about managing constant micro-adjustments. Even when you stand motionless, tiny muscles in the ankles and hips are firing to keep you upright. With age, those adjustments slow unless they are trained.

Exercises such as the “Knee Lift with Breeze Arms” highlight this beautifully. The act of lifting one knee, even just a few inches, forces the standing leg to stabilize. Adding gentle arm sweeps challenges coordination, making balance dynamic rather than rigid. You aren’t just learning to stand still—you’re learning to remain stable while in motion.

The Body as a Bridge

The body connects breath and balance into a single practice. Without the body, breath stays in the chest; without breath, the body stiffens; without balance, the body can’t trust itself to move. This interconnectedness is why exercises in this chapter use flowing imagery—“Sky Window Reach” or “Heart-Softening Wing”—to remind you that no part works alone.

The “Energy Ball Circle,” for example, coordinates arm spirals with steady breathing and a soft bend in the knees. It trains upper and lower body to move in sync while the breath keeps pace. The outcome isn’t just stronger arms or looser shoulders—it’s a nervous system that feels organized, a body that feels aligned, and a breath that feels natural.

Everyday Examples of Harmony

Think about climbing stairs while carrying groceries. Your body shifts weight from step to step, arms balance the load, and breath fuels the effort. If one part falters—if the breath shortens or the step wobbles—the task feels harder and less safe.

Or picture reaching up to close a window. Your arm rises, your spine lengthens, your feet anchor into the ground, and your breath helps stabilize the stretch. Without coordination, the movement might feel jerky or unsteady. With harmony, it feels smooth, almost effortless.

The Psychological Effect

Bringing breath, body, and balance together also affects the mind. People often describe feeling "centered" after these practices. That isn't a vague idea—it's the result of nervous system regulation. Deep breathing lowers heart rate, gentle movement reduces muscular tension, and practicing balance boosts confidence. The combination creates a sense of internal harmony that carries into daily life.

This psychological shift matters. Fear of falling, for instance, can sometimes cause more instability than physical weakness itself. By practicing controlled, harmonious movements, you not only strengthen your body but also retrain your mind to trust it again.

Building a Lasting Practice

The exercises in this chapter may look simple, but their impact compounds over time. Each spiral, reach, or cross-step is like a rehearsal for real life. The body learns to move smoothly, the breath becomes a steady partner, and balance feels less like a test and more like second nature. When these elements unite, harmony is no longer just an idea—it's a lived experience, present in every step you take.

Knee Lift with Breeze Arms

Duration: 1–2 minutes
Repetitions: 4–6 lifts per leg

Steps

- Stand tall with feet hip-width apart, knees relaxed.
- Shift weight gently to the left foot.
- Lift the right knee slightly while raising arms outward like a breeze.
- Lower arms and foot back to starting position.
- Repeat on the opposite side, alternating smoothly.

Goal

This pose improves balance, strengthens legs, and connects arm flow with gentle leg movement.

Safety tips: Keep lifts low; use a chair or wall for support if balance feels unsteady.

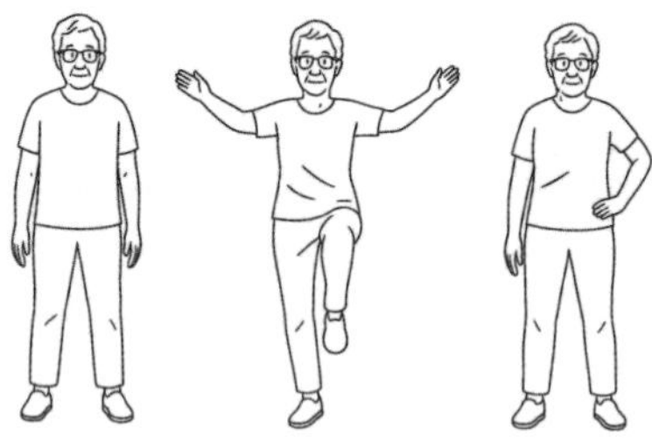

Sky Window Reach

Duration: 1–2 minutes
Repetitions: 4–6 reaches

Steps

- Stand with feet shoulder-width apart, knees soft.
- Hold hands together at chest height, palms facing out.
- Inhale as you open arms outward like opening a window.
- Exhale as you bring hands gently back together.
- Keep shoulders relaxed throughout the movement.

Goal

This pose opens the chest, encourages deep breathing, and promotes upper-body mobility.

Safety tips: Avoid overstretching; keep movements slow and comfortable.

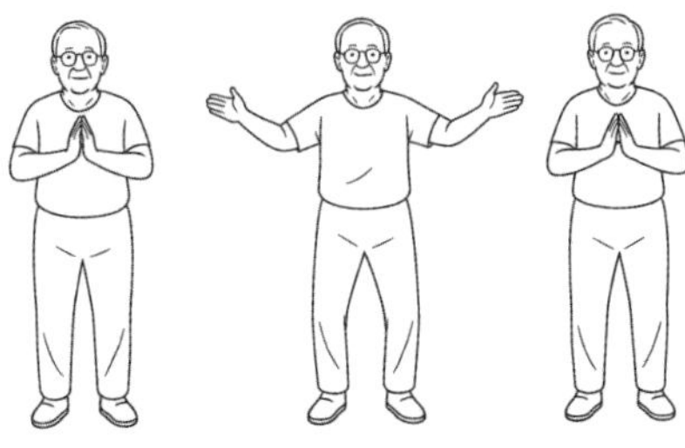

Energy Ball Circle

Duration: 1–2 minutes
Repetitions: 6–8 circles

Steps

- Stand with feet hip-width apart, knees relaxed.
- Hold hands in front of the belly as if cradling a ball.
- Move hands together in a slow circular motion to the right.
- Circle gently back to the left, keeping the ball shape.
- Breathe steadily as arms move.

Goal

This pose builds coordination, relaxes shoulders, and connects breath with flowing circular movement.

Safety tips: Keep circles small; avoid twisting too far at the waist.

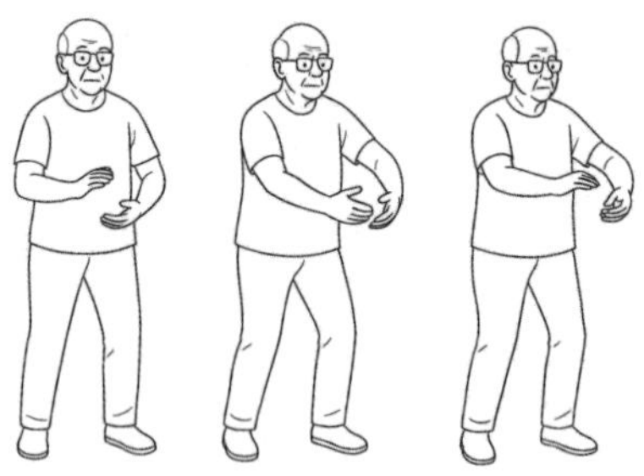

Spiral Palm Release

Duration: 1–2 minutes
Repetitions: 6–8 spirals

Steps

- Stand with feet shoulder-width apart, knees soft.
- Raise hands in front of the chest, palms facing out.
- Spiral palms outward slowly as if releasing tension.
- Draw hands back in gently to the center.
- Repeat with smooth, flowing motion.

Goal

This pose eases tension in wrists and arms, supports coordination, and creates a calming spiral flow.

Safety tips: Keep wrist spirals gentle; avoid overstretching arms.

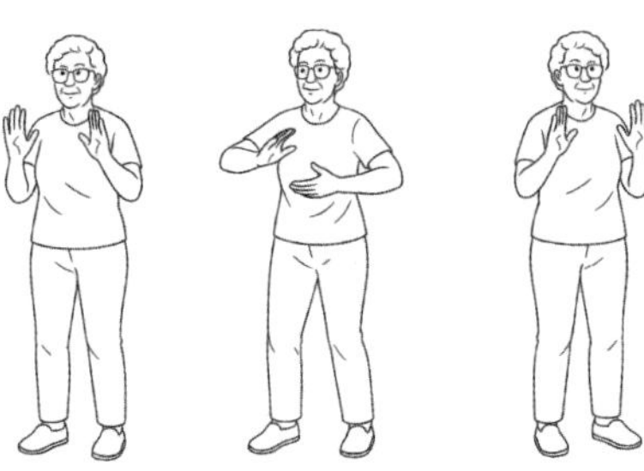

Weaving Cross-Step

Duration: 1–2 minutes
Repetitions: 4–6 steps each side

Steps

- Stand with feet hip-width apart, knees relaxed.
- Step the right foot gently across in front of the left.
- Bring arms across the body in a weaving motion.
- Return to center and repeat with the opposite foot.
- Continue alternating sides in a flowing rhythm.

Goal

This pose improves coordination, strengthens legs, and trains balance through gentle cross-steps.

Safety tips: Keep steps small and controlled; use a chair or wall nearby for balance.

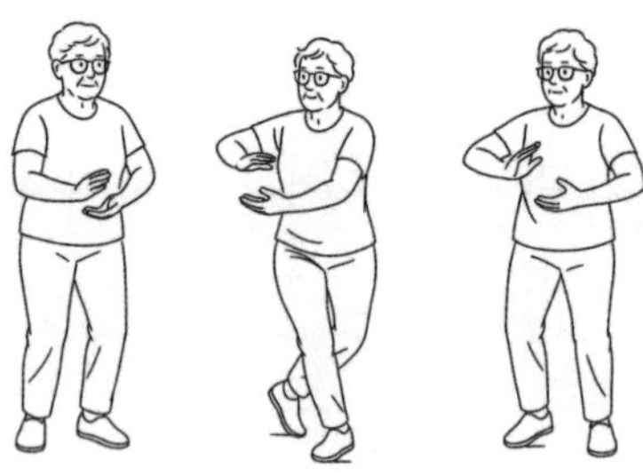

Leg Pendulum Swing

Duration: 1–2 minutes
Repetitions: 6–8 swings per leg

Steps

- Stand tall with feet hip-width apart, holding a chair or counter if needed.
- Shift weight to the left foot.
- Swing the right leg gently forward and back like a pendulum.
- Keep movements slow and small.
- Switch sides and repeat.

Goal

This pose loosens hips, strengthens legs, and supports balance with gentle swinging motion.

Safety tips: Keep swings low; hold onto support for safety.

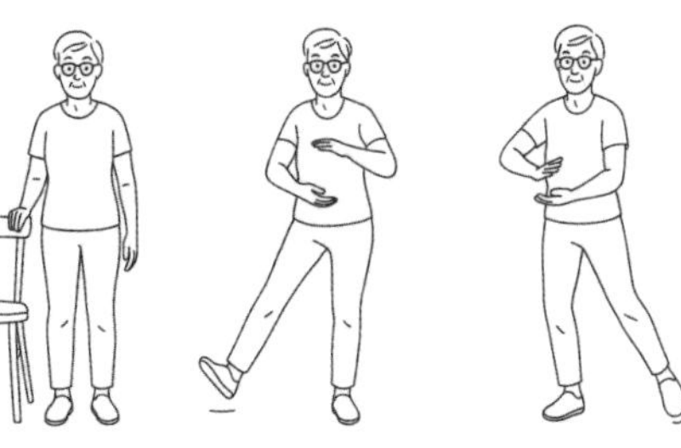

Heart-Softening Wing

Duration: 1–2 minutes
Repetitions: 4–6 times

Steps

- Stand with feet shoulder-width apart, knees soft.
- Bring palms together at chest height.
- Inhale as you open arms outward slowly like wings.
- Exhale as you bring palms gently back together.
- Keep chest lifted and shoulders relaxed.

Goal

This pose opens the chest, promotes relaxation, and encourages calm, mindful breathing.

Safety tips: Avoid raising arms higher than comfortable; move within easy range.

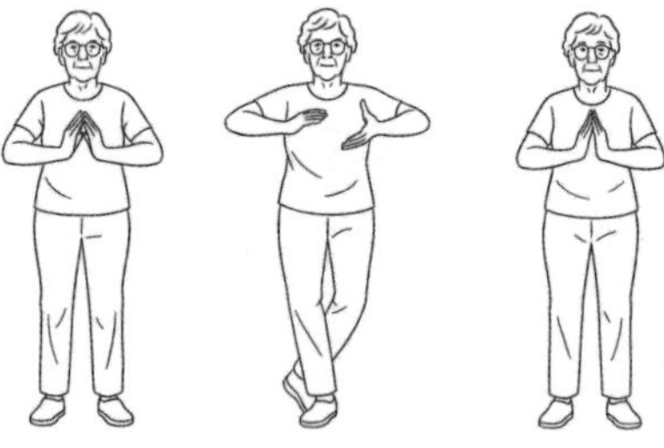

CONCLUSION

KEEP THE GAINS & KEEP GOING

Your 15-Minute Lifetime Plan

If there's one question that comes up again and again, it's this: *"How much do I really need to practice to keep the benefits?"* The good news is that you don't have to spend hours every day to maintain balance, strength, and calm. Fifteen minutes, done consistently, is enough to create lasting results. Think of it as brushing your teeth—not a grand workout, but a daily act of maintenance that keeps everything working smoothly.

Why 15 Minutes Works

Tai chi isn't about pushing your limits; it's about reinforcing patterns of posture, breath, and attention. These patterns are like grooves in the brain and body. Once carved, they only need regular use to stay strong. Research from Harvard Medical School has shown that even short sessions of tai chi, practiced several times a week, improve balance, reduce fall risk, and ease anxiety.

Fifteen minutes also fits into real life. It's short enough to do while waiting for dinner to cook, before bed, or as a morning ritual with your first cup of tea. For many seniors, the barrier isn't ability but time and energy. A quarter of an hour feels possible, even on a busy or low-energy day.

Structuring the 15 Minutes

A balanced routine has three parts: warm-up, flow, and close.

- **Warm-Up (3–4 minutes):** Gentle shoulder rolls, slow neck turns, and

light weight shifts. This prepares joints and signals to the mind that it's time to focus.
- **Flow (8–10 minutes):** A handful of tai chi movements practiced slowly and continuously. You don't need a long sequence; repeating two or three forms with mindful breath is more valuable than rushing through many.
- **Close (2 minutes):** Finish with quiet breathing, arms resting by the sides or palms over the belly. This seals the practice and leaves you calmer than when you began.

Over time, you may discover your own rhythm. Some prefer more warm-up, others extend the flow. The point is to make the plan repeatable and enjoyable.

Daily Life Integration

Fifteen minutes doesn't have to happen all at once. You can divide it into smaller chunks: five minutes after breakfast, five minutes mid-afternoon, and five minutes before bed. This approach is especially helpful for those managing conditions like arthritis, where shorter sessions reduce fatigue.

Everyday tasks can also serve as mini-practice. Standing at the sink, shift weight gently from one foot to the other. While waiting for the kettle to boil, practice "Floating Arms" with your breath. These moments add up and reinforce the same skills cultivated in your formal 15 minutes.

Examples from Real People

A retired nurse in her seventies found that practicing before bed improved her sleep. "Fifteen minutes of tai chi works better for me than a glass of wine or a pill," she said. Another man recovering from knee surgery chose mornings for his practice, saying, "It loosens me up for the whole day, like oiling a hinge."

These stories highlight that the plan is not rigid. The best schedule is the one you can keep.

Making It a Lifetime Habit

Habits stick when they're simple, rewarding, and tied to daily routines. Placing practice at the same time each day—before breakfast, after a walk, or before bed—anchors it. Many people also find that using a dedicated spot in the living room or garden helps; the space itself becomes a cue to move.

The reward is not distant. After just 15 minutes, most people feel calmer, looser, and steadier. That immediate feedback reinforces the habit more effectively than promises of long-term health.

Tai chi does not demand marathons of effort. It asks for steady attention, given a little each day. Fifteen minutes is enough to keep the gains you've made and carry them forward for a lifetime.

When and How to Progress Safely

In tai chi, progress doesn't mean moving faster or pushing harder. It means moving with greater ease, stability, and awareness. The beauty of the practice is that it can grow with you, whether you are just beginning or have years of experience. But like any physical activity, progress must be gradual and mindful, especially for older adults or anyone managing health conditions.

Knowing You're Ready to Progress

The first sign you're ready to take the next step is consistency. If you can practice your current routine comfortably for a few weeks without feeling unusually sore or fatigued, you're ready to add something new. Another sign is curiosity: if the movements start to feel familiar and you're eager for a new challenge, that's your body and mind telling you they're prepared.

For example, a participant who once needed a chair for balance may notice they rarely use it anymore. That's a natural cue to try a few movements without support. Similarly, if you can stand longer without fatigue, you may be ready to extend your practice time by five minutes.

Safe Ways to Increase Intensity

Progress can happen in many ways, not just by adding time. Consider these options:

- **Depth of Movement:** Bend the knees slightly more during weight shifts, always staying pain-free.
- **Repetition:** Instead of learning new movements right away, repeat familiar ones with slower, more controlled transitions.
- **Balance Challenges:** Try lifting one foot a little higher, or hold a stance for a few extra seconds.
- **Breath Coordination:** Focus more deeply on matching breath with each motion, which builds both awareness and calm.

The key is to change just one variable at a time. That way, you know what your body is responding to, and you avoid overwhelming yourself.

Listening to Warning Signs

Progress should never come at the cost of safety. Sharp pain, dizziness, or shortness of breath are signs to pause immediately. Muscle soreness after a new challenge can be normal, but joint pain that lingers is not. Many people mistake determination for progress, but in tai chi, patience is the greater strength.

A man in his early seventies once said, "I thought pushing through pain would make me stronger. Instead, it just kept me from showing up the next day." His lesson was that moving consistently, even at a lighter intensity, built more strength over time than sporadic overexertion.

Adding Variety Without Losing Focus

Some practitioners want to expand their routine by learning longer tai chi forms. This can be enriching, but it's not necessary for progress. Repeating a short sequence daily offers just as much benefit for balance, memory, and coordination.

If variety helps keep motivation high, you might alternate between seated practice one day and standing practice the next. Or you could practice in different environments—indoors one day, in the garden the next—to train balance under changing conditions.

What matters is not the complexity of the moves but the quality of attention you bring to them.

Progress Over Months, Not Days

Tai chi operates on a long timeline. Gains in stability, sleep, or energy often reveal themselves slowly, sometimes only when you look back months later. That's why keeping a journal or using a scorecard, as described earlier, can be so powerful. It makes gradual change visible.

Think of progress like a tree growing: you don't notice each millimeter, but one day you realize the trunk is stronger and the branches reach higher. In the same way, small daily improvements add up to lasting change.

Respecting Individual Limits

Everyone's path looks different. One person may increase practice time quickly, while another may stay at 15 minutes for years and still thrive. Some may focus on strength, others on breath or meditation. Comparing progress to others is less helpful than noticing your own small steps forward.

Safety, in the end, is not about holding yourself back—it's about creating the conditions to keep going. Tai chi is a lifetime practice, and the safest way to progress is to let the body lead, step by steady step.

Troubleshooting Common Hurdles

Even with the best intentions, practice rarely moves in a straight line. Some days your balance feels solid, other days your legs wobble like jelly. Sometimes the hardest part is not the movements themselves but the little roadblocks that get in the way. Recognizing these hurdles—and having strategies to handle them—keeps your practice alive and sustainable.

"I Don't Have Enough Time"

Time is the most common excuse, yet tai chi doesn't demand hours. Fifteen minutes is enough, and even five minutes is better than nothing. If a full session feels overwhelming, break it into smaller chunks: a few minutes after breakfast, a few before bed. One widower I worked with practiced while waiting for his coffee to brew. By the time the pot was done, he had already completed his warm-up.

The trick is reframing practice as part of daily life, not an extra chore. Folding tai chi into routines—standing at the sink, walking to the mailbox—removes the time barrier altogether.

"I Feel Awkward Doing the Movements"

Learning something new as an adult can feel humbling. The arms don't flow, the steps feel clumsy, and the names of movements sound mysterious. This awkwardness is not failure—it's the brain rewiring itself. Studies on motor learning show that coordination improves with repetition, not perfection on day one.

One group of seniors in a community center joked about feeling like "drunken cranes" in their first month. By the third month, they laughed again—but this time at how far they'd come. The message: awkwardness is part of the process, and it always passes.

"I Lose My Balance and Get Nervous"

Fear of falling is real, especially for those who've had one before. Tai chi helps by training balance, but until confidence builds, supports are your friend. Practicing near a wall, counter, or sturdy chair gives reassurance. Over time, as stability improves, you'll notice needing the support less often.

A veteran recovering from a hip replacement admitted, "At first, my counter was my best friend. Now, it's just there in case I need it, which I rarely do." Safety first, progress second.

"I Can't Remember the Sequence"

Tai chi forms can seem long and complicated. Forgetting the order often frustrates beginners, but the truth is you don't need to remember everything perfectly. Focusing on a handful of movements practiced slowly offers the same benefits as a full sequence.

Some people keep a simple note card with three or four movements written down. Others record their instructor on a phone and follow along at home. The point is not memorization but regular practice. As one teacher said, "Better to do three movements daily than thirty movements once a month."

"My Joints Hurt After Practice"

Mild muscle soreness can be normal, but sharp or lingering joint pain is a sign something needs adjusting. Often the issue is going too deep in the knees or locking the joints. Small changes—like reducing the bend, moving more slowly, or practicing seated—can make a big difference.

A woman with knee arthritis once said, "I thought I had to squat low to do it right. Once I learned to stay higher, the pain stopped—and I actually enjoyed it." Listening to your body is part of tai chi itself.

"I Get Bored"

Repetition builds skill, but it can also test patience. If boredom strikes, add variety without losing the essence. Try practicing outdoors, using music, or inviting a friend to join. Some enjoy alternating seated and standing sessions, or experimenting with imagery—imagining the arms as waves or clouds.

In Hong Kong parks, entire groups practice the same simple form daily, yet they stay engaged because it becomes a social ritual. The body moves, the mind calms, and the community connection keeps it fresh.

Turning Hurdles Into Part of the Practice

Every hurdle—time, memory, fear, discomfort—is not just an obstacle but a teacher. Each one offers a chance to adapt, to listen more closely, and to reshape the practice so it works for you. In that sense, troubleshooting is not outside the tai chi practice. It is the practice.

Next Steps: Community, Music & Joy

Tai chi may begin as an individual practice, but it often blossoms into something larger—connection, rhythm, and even joy. Once the basics feel familiar, many people find that sharing practice with others, adding music, or simply approaching it with playfulness deepens the experience in surprising ways.

Finding Community

Practicing alone has benefits, but tai chi in a group adds a special dimension. Moving in unison with others creates a sense of belonging, a quiet reminder that you're part of something larger. Research from social health studies shows that group activities reduce loneliness, lower depression scores, and even improve physical adherence to exercise routines.

Senior centers, local YMCAs, and parks often host tai chi classes, some tailored specifically to older adults. Many public libraries and cultural associations also list community programs. For those in rural areas or with limited mobility, online classes can offer connection, with live sessions allowing for interaction.

A retired teacher once remarked, "When I practice alone, I feel calmer. When I practice in class, I feel alive." Both experiences matter, and alternating between them can keep motivation strong.

Music as a Companion

Traditional tai chi is often practiced in silence, but music can be a powerful partner. Gentle instrumental pieces—flute, harp, soft piano, or nature sounds—help set a pace and soothe the nervous system. Music transforms the space, making even a small living room feel like a calm studio.

Some practitioners enjoy using familiar songs, associating each track with specific movements. Others prefer ambient sounds, like waves or rainfall, to encourage fluidity. The key is not volume but tone: music should support, not overpower, the breath and movement.

A study in geriatric rehabilitation noted that seniors who paired tai chi with calming music reported greater enjoyment and were more likely to continue the practice long-term. Rhythm and melody provide cues that guide the body without needing mental effort.

Joy in the Practice

Tai chi does not have to be solemn. In fact, playfulness often makes it more sustainable. Some groups incorporate light humor—naming movements in their own way or practicing outdoors where passersby can join spontaneously. Others bring grandchildren into the routine, turning tai chi into a multigenerational activity.

Joy also arises from small personal rituals. One woman in her eighties always lit a lavender candle before practice, saying it made her feel like she was “stepping into a sanctuary.” Another enjoyed practicing barefoot in her garden, feeling the grass under her feet as part of the meditation.

Building Your Next Chapter

Once tai chi becomes a habit, it can expand in many directions. You might join seasonal events, like World Tai Chi Day in April, where practitioners across the globe move together in public parks. You might explore cultural aspects, learning the history or philosophy behind the practice. Or you might simply keep deepening your personal routine, letting community, music, and joy weave into it naturally.

The next steps are not about scaling up difficulty but about broadening experience. Whether you connect with others, add rhythm, or infuse your practice with lightheartedness, tai chi grows with you. It’s not just about moving the body—it’s about keeping the spirit engaged.

YOUR EXCLUSIVE BONUSES

Your Guided Video Playlist

Sometimes, reading instructions and looking at illustrations is all you need. But other times, it feels even better to *see the movements in action*. To make your practice more accessible and inspiring, I've prepared a special video playlist created by some of the world's most respected Tai Chi teachers for seniors. These experts demonstrate each movement slowly, safely, and with the kind of clarity that makes you feel like you're right there in the class with them.

Watching the flow of their gestures, the calm rhythm of their breath, and the gentle alignment of posture can give you extra confidence as you practice. You'll notice small details—like the way the hands soften, or how the knees stay relaxed—that are sometimes easier to grasp visually than through text. Think of it as having your own personal teachers on screen, ready to guide you at any time, in your own space.

Scan the QR code now to unlock your private playlist and let the world's leading Tai Chi experts guide you step by step. Your practice will feel lighter, clearer, and more connected from the very first session.

Your Free Bonus Downloads

Unlock two helpful companion resources—free for readers of this book.

Bonus #1 — Quick-Start Program (7 Days to Confidence)

A simple, 10–15 minute-a-day plan to help you begin with calm and clarity. You'll get day-by-day focus points, gentle movements, and safety tips so you can build balance, mobility, and peace of mind—one small step at a time.

Bonus #2 — Printable Routine Guides (Step-by-Step Cues You Can Hold in Your Hand)

Clean, easy-to-follow practice sheets with posture and breathing cues, chair-supported options, a 10-minute daily flow, an evening wind-down, a complete seated routine, and a weekly progress tracker to help you stay consistent.

Point your phone's camera at the QR code and tap the link that appears. Download both bonuses in seconds, print what you need, and keep your practice steady, safe, and stress-free—starting now.